ASTHMA SURVIVAL

Other books by Robert S. Ivker, D.O.

Sinus Survival
Arthritis Survival
The Self-Care Guide to Holistic Medicine
Thriving

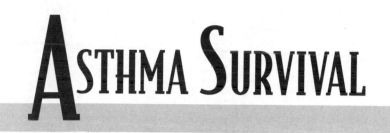

ASTHMA SURVIVAL

THE HOLISTIC MEDICAL TREATMENT PROGRAM FOR ASTHMA

ROBERT S. IVKER, D.O.
and TODD NELSON, N.D.

Jeremy P. Tarcher/Putnam
a member of Penguin Putnam Inc.
NEW YORK

Every effort has been made to ensure that the information contained in this book is complete and accurate. However, neither the publisher nor the author is engaged in rendering professional advice or services to the individual reader. The ideas, procedures, and suggestions contained in this book are not intended as a substitute for consulting with your physician. All matters regarding your health require medical supervision. Neither the author nor the publisher shall be liable or responsible for any loss, injury, or damage allegedly arising from any information or suggestion in this book.

Most Tarcher/Putnam books are available at special quantity discounts for bulk purchase for sales promotions, premiums, fund-raising, and educational needs. Special books or book excerpts also can be created to fit specific needs. For details, write Putnam Special Markets, 375 Hudson Street, New York, NY 10014.

Jeremy P. Tarcher/Putnam
a member of
Penguin Putnam Inc.
375 Hudson Street
New York, NY 10014
www.penguinputnam.com

Library of Congress Cataloging-in-Publication Data

Ivker, Robert S.
    Asthma survival : the holistic medical treatment program
for asthma / Robert S. Ivker and Todd Nelson.
        p.   cm.
    Includes index.
    ISBN 1-58542-124-3
    1. Asthma—Popular works.   2. Holistic medicine.
I. Nelson, Todd.   II. Title.

    RC591 .I95   2001   2001033210
    616.2'38—dc21

Printed in the United States of America

10 9 8 7 6 5 4 3 2 1

This book is printed on acid-free paper. ∞

To James, my nephew and godson,
and all children suffering the physical symptoms
and emotional causes of asthma

ACKNOWLEDGMENTS

I am most grateful to Phyllis Grann for choosing to include *Asthma Survival* as one of the five titles in the Tarcher/Putnam Survival Guide series. Although I had covered this subject to some extent in the third edition of *Sinus Survival,* asthma was clearly not the focus of the book. Researching and writing this book has been one of the most exciting experiences of my thirty-year medical career. But I could not have completed the job without the support and valuable contributions from my literary agent, Gail Ross; my publisher, Joel Fotinos; my editor, Mitch Horowitz, and his assistant, Allison Sobel; my coauthors of *The Self-Care Guide to Holistic Medicine,* Bob Anderson and Larry Trivieri; my friend and sponsor of the New Zealand trip, Bryce Brown; my allergy/asthma consultant, Bill Silvers; and my wife, Harriet.

Most of all I am deeply indebted to my coauthor, Todd Nelson. It was a pleasure to collaborate with him on this project. The synthesis of our nearly fifty years of clinical experience in treating patients with asthma produced this unique holistic approach. And the process of jointly creating this book, and *Arthritis Survival* before it, has not only solidified our professional relationship but has also inspired a lifelong friendship.

CONTENTS

INTRODUCTION: ASTHMA SURVIVAL

"Only when we are sick of our sickness shall we cease to be sick."

LAO-TSU, from the *Tao Te Ching*

The Asthma Survival story began with asthma's inclusion in the third edition of *Sinus Survival* in 1995. As a respiratory illness, asthma's causes and treatment are very similar to those of chronic sinusitis. Yet during the past twenty years the incidence of asthma has risen from 6 million in 1980 to more than 17 million in 1999, making it the eighth most common chronic ailment in America. Due to this dramatic increase, the corresponding concern triggered by more people (especially children) dying every year from asthma, and the recent advances made in our understanding of this disease, a separate book on the subject is warranted.

During the past fourteen years, I have treated a number of very ill patients who came to me primarily because they were suffering with chronic sinusitis. About 20 percent of these people were also asthmatic and were already under a physician's care for this problem. Although the Sinus Survival Program we implemented to treat these patients was primarily focused on their sinusitis, nearly all of them experienced considerable improvement of their asthma as well. Some were able to completely taper off of all of their inhalers and have continued to be free of any symptoms of asthma, while others were able to maintain good control of their asthma on much less medication. In recent years, as asthma has become a more serious and prevalent problem, I have devoted more attention to the treatment of this frightening respiratory condition. That research has led me to a collaborative effort with my coauthor, Dr. Todd Nelson, with the Asthma Survival Program and this book is the outcome.

Just as with sinusitis, there are multiple contributing factors—air pollution, immune dysfunction, allergy (both airborne and food), stress—but asthma is typically far more challenging to cure. Why? My educated guess is that the emotional and relationship issues most often accompanying this condition are much deeper and more difficult to heal than those usually seen with either sinusitis or allergies. But there remains much to be learned about asthma—so much so that medical science is still in relative infancy when it comes to understanding its causes.

This was made blatantly clear to me in July 2000 when I was invited to New Zealand to give a series of Sinus Survival seminars and workshops. That spectacularly beautiful country in the South Pacific, with essentially no air pollution, has the second-highest incidence of asthma in the world, and no one seems to know why. For two weeks during the middle of their winter, as I traveled throughout the country I became a health investigator. I was intrigued with their respiratory health crisis—they also have the world's tenth-highest incidence of allergies, while sinusitis is rampant. The results of my intensive two-week research revealed a myriad of factors that have combined to create this epidemic: high exposure to ultraviolet light through the hole in the earth's ozone layer, which weakens immunity; extremely high intake of milk and dairy products; soil that is devoid of selenium, a potent antioxidant; perennial high mold and, in some areas, pollen counts too; central heating that rarely heats homes above the high fifties (Fahrenheit) during the winter months; a "low-touch" society that was inherited from their puritanical British ancestors. As you'll read in Chapter 5, the lack of physical bonding—that is, affection—between mother or father and asthmatic child is a frequent finding with asthmatics.

The trip to New Zealand served as a powerful reminder that every chronic disease represents a state of imbalance and disharmony. Whether it's asthma, arthritis, or heart disease, there is a restriction or obstruction in the flow of life-force energy through body, mind, and spirit that stems largely from *a deprivation of love.* Holistic medicine, based on the belief that *unconditional love is life's most powerful healer,* is the most effective method I've found for healing any chronic condition. Applying and practicing each aspect of the Asthma Survival Program will provide you with new opportunities for loving and nurturing yourself, as well as specific ways to care for your body, that in turn will rekindle your inherent life-force energy and facilitate healing.

This book is based on the model of holistic medical treatment for chronic disease that I originally developed in the bestselling book *Sinus Survival.* Both of these books describe a program of self-healing and optimal health that includes a comprehensive guide to therapeutic options for treating, preventing, and potentially curing your asthma, sinusitis, or allergies.

Holistic medicine is defined as *the art and science of healing that addresses the whole person—body, mind, and spirit. Holistic physicians use both conventional and alternative therapies to prevent and treat disease, but most important, to promote optimal health.* In the following chapters I will present information to help you treat, prevent, and heal your asthma as well as to experience optimal well-being. This will include:

- Symptoms and diagnosis
- Conventional medical treatment
- Risk factors and causes
- Holistic medical treatment and prevention, with recommendations for body, mind, and spirit (including *diet, nutritional supplements, herbs,* and specific *physical, psychological,* and *bioenergetic therapies*)

The primary objective of this book is to teach you how to **love, nurture,** and **rejuvenate the chronically inflamed and hypersensitive mucous membranes lining your lungs.** This *reactive air-*

way disease (the medical terminology for asthma) is limiting the ability of you, or someone close to you, to breathe freely and easily, and as a result is significantly diminishing the quality of your life. I'm assuming that's why you bought the book. But, in addition to reversing the symptoms of asthma, it will be possible for you to experience a condition of *holistic health*—to feel better than you have in many years, while you relieve the inflammation and swelling of the mucous membranes.

Bear in mind, as you begin to implement this holistic treatment program, that true healing is far greater than simply the absence of illness. The most effective way to cure any chronic illness is to *heal your life,* not just repair your physical dysfunction, which in your case is difficult breathing. Therefore, I strongly advise that you use most of the tools and information provided in Chapters 3, 4, 5, and 6—"Holistic Health: The Thriving Self-Test," "Healing Your Body," "Healing Your Mind," and "Healing Your Spirit"—and not just simply rely on the quick fix in Chapter 1. What you learn in the latter chapters will assist you in strengthening your immune system and increasing your awareness of the physical, environmental, mental, emotional, spiritual, and social factors that may be contributing to your asthma. The specific therapies provided in these chapters will then enable you to more permanently reverse the symptoms and prevent recurrences, rather than experience a temporary fix. *The holistic treatment of any chronic disease includes addressing and eliminating the multiple causes; adhering to a healthy diet; getting regular exercise; making affirmations, visualizations, emotional work, prayer, or meditation a part of your daily life; and creating intimate relationships.* As a result, you will become much more sensitive to what foods, thoughts, feelings, or people make you feel good, and those that make you feel more uncomfortable or even aggravate your asthma. You can begin your training as a healer of your asthma by initially following the recommendations in Chapter 1, "The Asthma Quick Fix"; gaining a greater understanding of what asthma is in Chapter 2; and taking the Thriving Self-Test in Chapter 3. Then you will be ready to start the Asthma Survival Program in Chapter 4.

WORKING WITH YOUR PHYSICIAN

Although this book is intended as a self-care guide to healing asthma and creating optimal wellness, I recognize that most people will read it while under the care of a physician. I recommend that you use the suggested therapies as a *complement* to the medical treatment you may already be receiving, and I urge you to inform your doctor that you are doing so. Nothing in this book contradicts conventional medical treatment, and *proper drug use under the guidance of your physician can be practiced safely in conjunction with the complementary therapies I provide, unless specifically stated.* Holistic physicians recognize that drugs and surgery play an important role in treating disease, and I have included a section on the conventional medical treatment for asthma. My therapeutic recommendations are based on the successful approaches that I, Todd Nelson, N.D. (the cocreator of the Asthma Survival Program), and many of our holistic medical colleagues use to treat asthma in our clinical practices. They are not the only ones that work, but simply those with which we had the most experience. By following these recommendations, over time you will experience considerable improvement in your asthmatic condition, with great potential for freeing yourself of this disabling condition and feeling healthier than you ever have before. The comprehensive focus on healing all of the life issues that may be contributing to your asthma lies at the heart of the practice of holistic medicine and is the essence of the term *self-care.*

WORKING ON YOUR OWN

If you are not already under a physician's care, you might try starting with the holistic therapies on your own, unless otherwise indicated, and see how you feel after two months, before deciding to use conventional treatment or finding a holistic physician. And if you have been treated conventionally and conclude, after careful consideration and consultation with your physician, that the liabilities of the conventional treatment (such as dependency or unpleasant side effects from medication) outweigh their potential benefits, then commit solely to the holistic approach presented in the book, or take steps to find a holistic physician. One of the advantages of holistic medicine is that its combined use of complementary and conventional therapies often makes it possible to use lower dosages of medications to good effect, thereby minimizing harmful side effects.

HOLISTIC PHYSICIANS

If you are suffering from asthma (or any other chronic disease) or trying to improve the quality of your life, you may want the support of a holistic physician. You can find one in your area by contacting the American Holistic Medical Association (AHMA) on their website, www.holisticmedicine.org., to obtain their Physician Referral Directory. This list includes both physician members (M.D.s and D.O.s) and associate members (holistic practitioners other than M.D.s and D.O.s). The best resource for a referral to a *board-certified* holistic physician is the American Board of Holistic Medicine (ABHM). In December 2000, the ABHM administered the first certification examination in holistic medicine to nearly 300 physicians, setting a new standard for quality health care in America. To locate a board-certified holistic physician (M.D. or D.O.) near your home, contact the ABHM at 425-741-2996.

PROFESSIONAL COMPLEMENTARY THERAPIES

The discipline of holistic medicine includes the prudent use of both conventional Western medicine and professional care alternatives, such as *Ayurveda, acupuncture, behavioral medicine, Chinese medicine, chiropractic, energy medicine, environmental medicine, homeopathy, naturopathic medicine, nutritional medicine,* and *osteopathic medicine.* Chapters 4, 5, and 6 include mention of each of these therapies, which have been scientifically verified as appropriate professional care treatment for asthma. To learn more about these therapies, see the Resource Guide, which lists the primary organizations that oversee each of these therapies and provide a listing of practitioners nationwide. Each of them is also described in the appendix of *The Self-Care Guide to Holistic Medicine,* which I coauthored with Robert A. Anderson, M.D. (the president of the ABHM), and Larry Trivieri, Jr. That book also presents the holistic medical treatment for sixty-five of America's most common ailments.

CHARTING YOUR PROGRESS

One way to monitor the progress of your holistic treatment program for asthma is to evaluate your physical symptoms on a weekly basis. You can do so by using a chart similar to the Symptom Chart shown on page 62. This is an example of a Respiratory Disease symptom chart, and lists the most common symptoms you may experience if you suffer from asthma, sinusitis, allergies, or bronchitis. If you experience symptoms not included on this list, then add them in the left-hand column and rank them from 1 (worst) to 10 (best or no symptoms) on a weekly basis. You can also uncover possible emotional factors that are contributing to your condition by similarly ranking your emotional stress level each week. You should be able to graphically correlate higher stress with worsening physical symptoms. The same is often true with dietary factors. Also keep track of the medications, herbs, nutritional supplements, and other remedies you are using at the bottom of the chart. *Note: The vitamins, herbs, and supplements recommended in Chapter 4 are available in most health food stores, and through Thriving Health Products. The suggested dosages are based on those that I, Todd Nelson, and our holistic colleagues have used extensively in our clinical practices. These dosages may vary from the suggestions of your own personal holistic physician.*

By using the Symptom Chart you can more easily evaluate your progress and better determine what works for you and what doesn't. (Remember, each of us is a unique individual, with specific needs and requirements in order to be healthy.) As you practice using this chart you'll become quite adept at the early recognition of dietary, environmental, and emotional factors that aggravate your asthma, and be able to quickly respond with an effective therapy. The better you become at listening to your body, mind, and spirit, the more effectively you will be able to *prevent* recurrences of your condition. This art, science, and discipline is the basis for the practice of both holistic and preventive medicine. As you continue your training you will develop into a highly skilled self-healer. Although you may be starting out suffering with asthma, remember that the greater your *enjoyment* of this life-changing challenge, the better your results will be.

This book is meant to enlighten and educate you: You'll learn why you've had difficulty breathing for so long, and what you can do to improve that condition. But for the Asthma Survival Program to make a profound difference in your life, you'll need to give yourself a gentle but firm push in the direction of optimal health—a condition of high energy and vitality, creativity, peace of mind, self-awareness, self-acceptance, passion, and intimacy. The critical ingredients for your success are a heightened *awareness* of your needs and desires (What do want your life to be like?); a *commitment* to providing them for yourself; the *time* required to incorporate new healthy habits into your life; and the *discipline* to stay on your course in spite of difficulty breathing and fear. These are the essential factors in learning to love and nurture yourself, and especially the mucous membranes lining your lungs. And it is also the primary objective of this holistic medical treatment program.

If you are willing to make the commitment, this program will enable you to *heal yourself of asthma*. Although you might still have an occasional attack of wheezing, you will no longer experience chronic shortness of breath, significant disability, or daily dependence on inhalers and bronchodilators. More important, you will understand why the wheezing attack occurs, have the tools to treat it quickly, and avoid the terrifying experience of fighting to breathe for a prolonged period of time. But the most significant aspect of your healing process is that you will almost always learn or relearn a valuable lesson through your wheezing that helps to *prevent* subsequent attacks.

Although optimal health requires a commitment to a lifelong healing *process,* we live in an age of the quick fix. We've grown up believing that there's a fast and effortless solution to all of life's hardships. And if there is not such a miracle available today, it won't be long before science and technology provide it. But to heal your dysfunctional lungs, while creating a balance of optimal well-being throughout every dimension of your life, requires a commitment to the Asthma Survival Program comparable to one you would make starting a new job. *Healing yourself is the most important work you'll ever do, and the greatest gift you'll ever receive.*

After two months of making a commitment to this program, you will probably be "surviving" quite well, with a significant improvement in your symptoms. If you can maintain and strengthen that commitment to yourself, within six months you will be healthier than you've been in years, and within one year you'll be experiencing a state of well-being you've never known before. The most important advice I can give you is to take your time, be gentle and accepting of yourself, and know that there are no mistakes—only lessons. Study diligently, listen attentively, be willing to take risks, and have fun while you're at it. It's definitely a challenge, but the rewards are unimaginable!

Rob Ivker
January 2001

Chapter 1

THE ASTHMA QUICK FIX

After just describing the Asthma Survival Program in the Introduction as a *healing process* and not a *quick fix,* you may be wondering about the title of this chapter. I realize that upon embarking on a life-changing program requiring a strong personal commitment, most people in our society would like a simple and safe way to take the initial step. To facilitate change, you must first diminish the resistance that may arise from the anticipation of how much time and expense you will need to invest in this program. You may also need to modify your attitude in approaching long-term dietary changes as well as taking dietary supplement pills on a regular basis. In addition, you might be confronting the fear of reducing and, hopefully, eliminating your inhalers, since you may have had unpleasant experiences with trying to do so in the past. That is perfectly understandable. Therefore, rather than trying to do everything at once, which for many people can also be a bit overwhelming, this chapter will offer you several options for more *gradually* introducing this holistic approach into your life while experiencing relatively rapid ***symptom improvement.***

The primary objective of the Asthma Survival Program and the holistic treatment for any chronic disease is to heal the specific part of the body that is not functioning properly. The method for correcting this physical dysfunction is for you to nurture not only the diseased part but your entire body along with your mind and spirit.

This healing process usually begins on the physical level, because the body provides the most immediate feedback, telling you what feels good and what makes you feel worse. But if you're feeling some degree of difficulty breathing all the time, it's not easy to determine what one intervention—an herb, dietary change, or air cleaner—is doing for you. It has usually taken many months or years to produce the conditions creating your ongoing asthmatic problem. Therefore, it will take some time for your body to function well enough on a consistent basis to begin to trust the signals and feedback it is giving you. By improving physically at the outset, you'll become much more aware of what you can do to heighten this feeling of well-being and what behaviors—what you're eating, too little or too much exercise, not enough sleep, specific stressors—make you feel worse. Over time you will learn to become your own best healer and develop reference points for what techniques work best for you. To speed the process of correcting the imbalances in your life, I have developed the initial **Physical** and **Environmental Health** Components of the Asthma Survival Program, which are summarized in this first chapter. It won't be effortless, but if you're committed to healing and curing your asthma, this is the most effective way to begin your new full-time job. This approach will enable you to feel better as quickly as possible. Chapters 2 through 6 will help you to understand *why* all of these recommendations are included and to better appreciate how they are helping to maintain and enhance your health.

I've found that if you stay on the complete regimen described in this chapter for at least four to eight weeks, you will usually be able to at least partially restore the physical imbalance and experience considerable and often dramatic improvement. You should also be able to decrease the use of your inhalers and oral medication. These physical and environmental health recommendations are outlined on the following pages in Tables 1.1 and 1.2, and are explained in more depth in Chapter 4. The improvement in your physical condition will usually provide the motivation to commit to and fully benefit from the Mind and Spirit Components of the Program while addressing all of the causes of your illness.

The practice of holistic medicine is based on loving yourself physically, environmentally, mentally, emotionally, spiritually, and socially. There is no quick fix in this lifetime process of experiencing optimal health. Since each of us is a unique individual, our prescription for *healing is based on self-awareness.* However, you can give yourself a jump start by closely following the majority of these initial recommendations, which work quite well for almost anyone.

In the tables that follow, I have placed **one asterisk** in the left margin next to the recommendations, vitamins, and supplements that should be started at the outset—**stage one. Two asterisks** denote the **second stage,** which you can begin three weeks later. The **third stage,** marked by **three asterisks,** begins after another three weeks. You always have the option of doing and taking everything right from the beginning or at any time of your choosing, and simply following the instructions in the table. The only risk that I'm aware of in starting out with the entire program is that it could feel a bit overwhelming and may be more challenging to *maintain* the new daily practices than if you gradually ease into it.

It is important to note that if you are working with a holistic physician or practitioner, he or she will probably want to establish some baseline pulmonary function tests (see page 38) *before* you begin any aspect of the Asthma Survival Program. These tests are an integral part of a comprehensive initial evaluation that your physician will need to help you design a more personalized treatment program.

Each of the different therapeutic options presented in the following tables will contribute some benefit. There is no single remedy or magic potion that will quickly cure asthma. However, most people who are interested in this program have been uncomfortable for many months, if not years. For them, taking two to four months to feel better than they have in a long time can be described as a *quick fix*.

After about two months of incorporating most of the physical and environmental health recommendations into your daily routine, you can begin the mental and emotional health components of the program, followed in another one to two months by spiritual and social health. These facets of the program will be described in Chapters 5 and 6. With each component you will be uncovering factors that have contributed to causing your asthma. Remember, the more often you experience a sense of physical well-being, the more acutely aware you'll become of what makes you feel good and what triggers your wheezing. This information initially will allow you to make healthier choices regarding what and how you're breathing, where and how you exercise, and what you eat and drink. Your diet will make a significant difference, but as you progress you'll find that what you eat may be less important than what's eating you! You'll soon realize that the latter four aspects of health—comprising the *mind* and *spirit* sections—require far less of your time but a deeper commitment and greater awareness than the recommendations for the *body*. However, the more you can work on these less tangible but potentially more immune-suppressing and -enhancing factors, the more you will be able to effectively *prevent* asthmatic attacks, *reduce* or eliminate your inhalers, and possibly *cure* yourself of asthma.

Before you begin implementing the Physical and Environmental Health Component, please take the Thriving Self-Test in Chapter 3 and the Candida Questionnaire and Score Sheet in Chapter 4. Your wellness score will help you to see where your life is unbalanced and what aspects of the Asthma Survival Program will require the bulk of your attention. If your candida score is above 120 (woman) or 80 (man), then I would consider candida as a probable cause of your asthma and recommend adding the Candida Treatment Program (Table 1.4) on page 21 to the rest of the physical and environmental recommendations right from the start. If your score is lower, then I'd wait at least four to six weeks and see how you feel after strictly adhering to the Physical and Environmental Health Components. Then, if there's no improvement, I would consider adding the treatment for candida. This treatment program is described in more depth in Chapter 4 beginning on page 102. I would also suggest reading Chapter 4, Healing Your Body, to have a better understanding of why the therapies in the following tables are used. Since many asthmatic attacks are triggered by the common cold, the Cold Treatment Program (Table 1.3) on page 20 is included. If you can quickly eliminate (or prevent) the cold, you can often avoid a flare-up of asthma.

Many of the products included in these tables that are not readily available at most health food stores can be obtained by referring to the Product Index at the end of the book.

Table 1.1

The Physical and Environmental Health Components of the *Asthma Survival Program* for Preventing and Treating *Asthma*

	PREVENTIVE MAINTENANCE	TREATING ASTHMA
★ Sleep (p. 199)	7–9 hrs/day; no alarm clock	8–10+ hrs/day
★ Breathing exercises (p. 86)	Practice 3 times/day for at least 5 to 10 min	
★ Negative ions or air cleaner (p. 71)	Continuous operation; use ions especially with air-conditioning.	Continuous operation
★★ Room humidifier, warm mist (p. 80); and ★★★ central humidifier (p. 81)	Use during dry conditions, especially in winter if heat is on and in summer if air conditioner is on.	Continuous operation
★ Saline nasal spray (SS spray) (p. 98)	Use daily, several times/day, especially with dirty and/or dry air.	
★ Steam Inhaler (p. 97)	Use as needed with dirty and/or dry air.	Use daily, 2–4×/day; (add SS eucalyptus oil)
★ Water, bottled or filtered (p. 91)	Drink ½ oz./lb. body weight; with exercise ⅔ oz./lb.	
★ Diet (p. 140) ★ Candida Diet (p. 125)	NLEP—increase fresh fruit, vegetables, whole grains, fiber; cayenne, ginger, onions, and garlic; decrease sugar, dairy, wheat, and alcohol; do food elimination to determine any food allergy.	
★ Exercise, preferably aerobic (p. 189)	Minimum 20–30 min, 3–5×/week; avoid outdoors if high pollution and/or pollen, and extremely cold temperatures.	No aerobic; moderate walking OK. Avoid outdoors if high pollution and/or pollen, and cold temperatures.

Table 1.2

Vitamins and Supplements for Preventing and Treating *Asthma*

	Adults		Children (Over 3 Yrs of Age)		Pregnancy	
	(★1) PREVENTIVE MAINTENANCE	TREATING ASTHMA	PREVENTION	TREATING ASTHMA	PREVENTION	TREATING ASTHMA
★ Vitamin C (polyas-corbate or ester C)	1,000–2,000 mg 3×/day	3,000–5,000 mg 3×/day	100–200 mg 3×/day	500–1,000 mg 3×/day	1,000 mg 2×/day	1,000 mg 4×/day
★ Vitamin E (natural d-alpha mixed tocopherols; avoid if soy-sensitive or use soy-free E)	400 IU 1 or 2×/d	400 IU 2×/d	50 IU 1 or 2×/d	200 IU 2×/d	200 IU 1×/d	200 IU 2×/d
★ Proantho-cyanidin (grape-seed extract)	100 mg 1 or 2×/d (on an empty stomach)	200 mg 3×/d (on an empty stomach)	—	100 mg 1×/d	—	100 mg 1×/d
★ Vitamin B$_6$	50 mg 2×/d	200 mg 2×/d	10 mg 1×/d	25 mg 1×/d	25 mg 1×/d	25 mg 2×/d
★ Vitamin B$_{12}$	500 mcg 1×/d sublingually	1000 mcg 1×/d (under tongue)	—	—	—	500 mcg 1×/d
(★2) Multivita-min	1 to 3×/d	1 to 3×/d	Pediatric multivitamin		Prenatal multivitamin with 800 mg folic acid	
★ Magne-sium glycinate, arginate, or aspartate	500 mg/d	500 mg/d 2–3×/d	150–250 mg/d	300 mg/d	500 mg/d	500 mg/d
★ Selenium	100–200 mcg/d	200 mcg/d	—	100 mcg/d	25 mcg/d	100 mcg 2×/d
★ (★3) Fish oils (Omega-3 fatty acids)	EPA: 400–600 mg 3×/d DHA: 300–500 mg/d		EPA: 200–300 mg 3×/d DHA: 100–200 mg/d		EPA: 400–600 mg 3×/d DHA: 300–500 mg/d	

	Adults			Children (Over 3 Yrs of Age)			Pregnancy	
★①	PREVENTIVE MAINTENANCE	TREATING ASTHMA	PREVENTION	TREATING ASTHMA		PREVENTION	TREATING ASTHMA	
★ Quercetin	—	1,000 mg 3–6×/day	—	250–500 mg 3×/day		—	—	
★ Bromelain	1,000 mg on empty stomach							
† Lobelia (tincture)	—	25 drops in mint tea every 3–4 hrs	—	12 drops in mint tea every 3–4 hrs		—	—	
★✪ Ephedra or Ma huang	—	12.5–25 mg 2 or 3×/d	—	5 mg 2×/d		—	—	
★ Ginkgo biloba	—	40 mg of 24% standardized extract 3×/d	—	20 mg of 24% standardized extract 3×/d		—	—	
★ Coleus forskohlii	—	25–50 mg of 18% standard-ized extract of forskolin 2–3×/d	—	12.5–25 mg of 18% standardized extract of forskolin 2–3×/d		—	—	
★ N-acetylcy-stein (NAC)	500 mg/d	500 mg 3×/d standardized extract 3×/d	—	300 mg 3×/d standardized extract 3×/d		—	500 mg 3×/d	
★ Glutathione	—	100 mg 3–4×/day	—	100 mg daily		—	—	
★ Garlic 4,000 mcg/ pill	1,200 mg/d	1,200–2,000 mg 3×/d	—	1,000 mg 3×/d		—	1,200 mg 3×/d	
★④ Acidoph-ilus (lacto-bacillus + bifidus)	½ tsp or 2 caps 2×/d	¼ tsp 2×/d	—	½ tsp or 2 caps 2×/d		—		
★ Grapefruit (citrus) seed extract (Nutribiotic)	—	100 mg 3×/d or 10 drops in water 3×/d	—	4 drops in water 2×/d		—	100 mg 3×/d or 10 drops in water 3×/d	
★⑥ Candida-Free	2 capsules 1 hour after meals 3×/d	—	—	—		—		

	Adults		Children (Over 3 Yrs of Age)		Pregnancy	
	PREVENTIVE MAINTENANCE	**TREATING ASTHMA**	**PREVENTION**	**TREATING ASTHMA**	**PREVENTION**	**TREATING ASTHMA**
★★ Beta carotene (food-derived with mixed carotenoids)	25,000 IU 1 or 2×/d	★7 25,000 IU 3×/d	5,000 IU 1 or 2×/d	10,000 IU 2×/d	25,000 IU 1×/d	25,000 IU 2×/d
★★ Zinc arginate	20–40 mg/d	40–60 mg/d	10 mg/d	10 mg 2×/d	25 mg/d	40 mg/d
★★ Calcium (citrate or hydroxyapatite)	1,000 mg/d; menopause: 1,500 mg/d	1,000 mg/d; menopause: 1,500 mg/d	600–800 mg/d from diet		1,200 mg/d	1,200 mg/d
★★★ Chromium picolinate	200 mcg/day	200 mcg/day	—	—	in prenatal multi-vitamin	
★★★ Pantothenic acid	250 mg/day	500 mg 3×/d	—	50 mg 2–3×/d	—	—
★★★ Hydrochloric acid	10–20 grains after protein meals					
★★★ Folic acid	800 mcg/d	add 1 to 5 mg/d if on oral steroids	—	—	—	—
★★★ ★8 Whole adrenal extract	250 mg/d	follow directions on bottle	—	—	—	—

Key to Tables 1.1 and 1.2

★1 Use the higher dosage on days of higher stress, less sleep, and increased air pollution.

★2 Dosage depends on brand.

★3 Use with caution for those with fish allergies and aspirin sensitivity.

★4 Use only if wheezing is a primary symptom, but do not use with high blood pressure.

★5 Use dairy-free acidophilus and bifidus A.M. and P.M. (empty stomach) for 3 wks at a time, following antibiotics and/or every few months as prevention for candidiasis.

★6 Use only if candida is suspected and take no longer than 2 months without supervision.

★7 Use this dosage for a maximum of 1 month.

★8 Use only if fatigue is a significant symptom or with a history of long-term steroid use.

★ Stage One—begin the program with these.

★★ Stage Two—take these after 3 weeks into the program, or earlier if you choose.

★★★ Stage Three—start these 6 weeks into the program, or sooner if you're comfortable with doing so.

Acute Treatment Options
(only under the supervision of a physician)

In *addition* to those listed in Table 1.2 under the "Treating Asthma" column.

- IV magnesium, alone or in "Meyers Cocktail," during an asthma attack
- IV vitamin C, 10–25 grams, at the onset of a cold (can potentially prevent both the cold and the asthmatic attack)
- IV B_{12}: 1,000 mcg weekly, or in accordance with Wright Protocol
- Glutathione, 400 mg/d, either orally or IV. (Recommend Tyler Encapsulations Recancostat for oral administration.)
- UltraInflamX (Metagenics)—an anti-inflammatory medical food powder used for therapeutic detoxification.

Table 1.3

Cold Treatment Program★

- Rest and get more sleep.
- Take vitamin C (in the form of ester C), between 15 and 20,000 mg in the first 24 hours; either 5,000 mg 3 or 4×/day or 2,000 mg every 2 hours, or 1,000 mg every waking hour; very gradually taper this dose over the next 3–5 days.
- Take vitamin A (kills viruses), 150,000 IU daily for 2–3 days; you can take 50,000 IU three times, then gradually taper over the next 2–3 days.
- Take Yin Chiao, a Chinese herb, 5 tablets 4 or 5×/day in the first 48 hours.
- Take garlic, eaten raw (one or two cloves a day) or in liquid or capsule form, 4,000 mcg (of allicin) per day.
- Take echinacea, or EchinOsha Blend® (combination of echinacea with osha root and other herbs), 1 dropperful in water 3–5×/day for 3–5 days; or 900 mg 4×/day. Do not take echinacea if you have an autoimmune disease like lupus, MS, or HIV.
- Take zinc gluconate lozenges, containing at least 13 mg, every 2 hours.
- Gargle with salt water.
- Use a saline nasal spray hourly, preferably the Sinus Survival Spray containing antiviral herbs.
- Take lots of warm or hot liquids; take ginger root or peppermint tea; you can include ginger, honey, lemon, cayenne, cinnamon, and a teaspoon of brandy.
- Take a hot bath and inhale steam, adding a few drops of eucalyptus, peppermint, and/or tea tree oil.
- Take the homeopathic *Aconitum* (monkshood).
- Eliminate dairy products, bread, concentrated fruit juices, and sugar. Eat lighter foods such as soups, stews, and steamed vegetables; eat less protein.

★ This treatment program is highly effective for diminishing both the duration and intensity of a cold, and works best the more quickly you respond to the first symptoms of a cold. They are usually a sore throat, fatigue, feeling weak or achy, mucus drainage, and possibly some sneezing.

Table 1.4

Candida Treatment Program ⍟1

- Candida diet—refer to Chapter 4.
- Antifungal medication (Rx)—Diflucan, Sporanox, or Nizoral.⍟2
- Antifungal homeopathic—Mycocan Combo, Aqua Flora, Candida-Away, and several others—an alternative to antifungal Rx.
- Latero-Flora (found in health food stores as Flora Balance)—2 capsules 20 min before breakfast.⍟3
- Acidophilus (*Lactobacillus acidophilus* and *bifidus,* Ethical Nutrients brand is best)—½ teaspoon or 2 caps 3×/day for adults and during pregnancy; ¼ teaspoon 3×/day for children over 3.⍟4
- Candida-Free—2 capsules 1 hour after meals.⍟5
- Garlic, eaten raw (one or two cloves a day) or in liquid, tablet, or capsule form, 4,000 mcg (of allicin) per day. (Metagenics Super Garlic 6000, Ethical Nutrients, or PhytoPharmika)
- Colon hydrotherapy (colonic) treatments.⍟6

Key to Candida Treatment Program

⍟1 To determine if you are a candidate for candida treatment, first take the Candida Questionnaire and Score Sheet in Chapter 4. If your total score is in the "Probably Yeast-Connected" range or higher (above 120 for women and 80 for men), then consider committing to the candida treatment if there is no improvement after 6 weeks on the Asthma Survival Program outlined in the preceding tables.

⍟2 Antifungal medication needs to be prescribed and monitored by a physician. If you are unable to find a physician willing to prescribe this, you can either find a holistic physician or consider taking an antifungal homeopathic, although they are not quite as effective as the medication. The higher your candida score, the more important it is to include an Rx or homeopathic (or both—the homeopathic can complement the Rx) in your treatment program. Expect some "die-off" effect with possible worsening of your symptoms within the first 2 weeks after beginning this medication, and with the homeopathic too. Recommended dosage for either of these three medications is 200 mg daily for 4 to 6 weeks, then every other day for 3 to 4 weeks.

⍟3 A beneficial bacteria that is effective in killing candida. Usual dosage is 2 capsules daily 20 min before breakfast for 2 or 3 months, then 1 capsule for an additional 2–3 months.

⍟4 Begin taking acidophilus at the outset of candida treatment. While restoring normal bacterial flora, it can also assist in detoxification, reducing toxic uptake during die-off, and shorten duration of treatment.

⍟5 Available through Thriving Health Products.

⍟6 Not absolutely necessary, but can speed your progress especially during the first month of treatment. To find a colon hydrotherapist, call the office of a holistic (M.D. or D.O.) or naturopathic (N.D.) physician, or a chiropractor.

Table 1.5

Natural Quick-Fix Symptom Treatment

Cough
Gargle, then drink lemon juice and honey (1:1) with a tablespoon of
  vodka (not with Candida) or a pinch of cayenne pepper.
Ginger tea
Wild cherry bark syrup
Bronchial drops (a homeopathic)
Sinus Survival Cough Syrup (with elderberry)
Licorice teas
Bronchoril Expectorant: 2 pills before meals for dry cough (Phyto
  Pharmika or Enzymatic Therapy brand)

Fatigue
Ginseng
Antioxidants, especially vitamin C
Folic acid
Vitamin B_{12}, 500 mcg 2×/day
Vitamin B_6, 75 to 100 mg/day
Pantothenic acid, 500 mg 1 or 2×/day
Meditation
Breathing exercises
Exercise
Sleep
Pace yourself between activity and rest
Rule out anemia

Headache
Adequate water intake
Negative air ions
Meditation
Breathing exercises
Steam
Eucalyptus oil
Acupressure/reflexology points
Hydrotherapy—alternate hot and cold shower
Garlic or horseradish (chew it)
Calcium/magnesium
Quercetin, 2 caps 3×/day
Ginkgo biloba, 40 mg 3×/day
Magnesium glycinate, 200 mg 2×/day
Feverfew avena, 20 drops 3×/day; or a standardized extract, 1 pill
  2×/day

Runny Nose
Adequate water intake
Saline spray every 1 to 2 hours
Ephedra (not with high blood pressure)
Freeze-dried Nettles, 1 cap 3×/day
Quercetin, 1,000 mg, 2 tabs 3×/day (on an empty stomach)—take
   with bromelain
Vitamin C, 6,000 to 10,000 mg/day or higher—take as ascorbate or
   Ester C

Sneezing
Adequate water intake
Acupressure/reflexology points
Freeze-dried Nettles, 2 caps 2–3×/day
Quercetin, 1,000 mg, 2 tabs 3×/day (on an empty stomach)—take
   with bromelain

Sore Throat
Gargle with lemon juice and honey (1:1)
Gargle with pinch of cayenne + 1 tsp salt in 8 oz water.
Licorice-based tea (Long Life, Traditional Medicinals, or Throat Coat)
Lozenges (Zand Eucalyptus, Holistic brand Propolis)
Zinc arginate, 30 mg 3×/day—begin with zinc gluconate lozenges
   for three days, then switch to arginate
Garlic, 2 caps 3×/day
Herbal throat spray—there are many good brands

Stuffy Nose
Adequate water intake
Hot tea with lemon
Hot chicken soup
Steam
Hydrotherapy (hot water from shower) or hot compresses
Eucalyptus oil
Horseradish
Anger release, especially punching
Acupressure/reflexology points
Massage
Orgasm
Exercise
Garlic
Onions
Cayenne pepper
Breathe Right™—External Nasal Dilator
No ice-cold drinks

No dairy
No gluten (wheat, rye, oats, barley)
Ephedra, 20 to 30 drops 4×/day for 2–3 days (max.)
Rule out allergies.
Papaya enzyme, 1 or 2 tablets 4×/day (dissolved in mouth)—use also
   for ear congestion, sinus congestion, and sinus pain
Sinupret, or Quanterra Sinus Defense (a combination of five herbs)

Wheezing

Breathing exercises
Ephedra, 12.5 to 25 mg or 2 or 3×/day (can increase heart rate and
   anxiety—don't use if you have high blood pressure)
Lobelia, 25 drops in mint tea every ½ to 1 hour (may cause nausea)
Coleus forskoli, 25–50 mg as 18% standardized extract 3x/day
   (Phyto Pharmica brand). No gluten grains or sulfites
No milk or dairy
Caffeine
Magnesium glycinate, citrate, or aspartate, 250 mg every 3 hours
Vitamin B_6, 200 mg 2x/day
Vitamin B_{12}, 500 mcg (sublingual) 2×/day
Vitamin C, 3,000 to 5,000 3×/day
Selenium, 200 mcg 1×/day
Onions

Chapter 2

WHAT IS ASTHMA? WHAT CAUSES IT? HOW DOES CONVENTIONAL MEDICINE TREAT IT?

Asthma is the most frightening and life-threatening of the common respiratory conditions. It is a chronic disease in which the lining of the airways in the lungs (bronchi and bronchioles) becomes inflamed, swollen, and produces extra mucus. As a result, the airways narrow, making it difficult to breathe. The most common symptoms are:

- Wheezing (a whistling or hissing sound as you exhale)
- Shortness of breath
- Feelings of tightness or constriction in the chest (like someone is squeezing your chest)
- Coughing

You may have all of these symptoms, some of them, or just one. Asthma symptoms are recurrent and can be mild or severe. Within the bronchi and bronchioles, the small airways, asthma causes:

1. Swelling of the respiratory mucosa lining the airway
2. Thicker and increased mucus secretion into the airway

3. Contraction of the smooth muscle lining the bronchiolar walls

These three obstructive changes occurring together leave very little room for air to pass through. In addition to airway *obstruction,* asthma is also characterized by airway *inflammation.* This, in turn, causes airway hyperresponsiveness, resulting in a heightened *sensitivity* to pollen, air pollution, tobacco smoke, mold, animal dander, the common cold, and cold and dry air.

The Centers for Disease Control and Prevention (CDC) estimated that in 1998, approximately 17.3 million people in the United States, or 6.4 percent of the population, self-reported having asthma. This represents more than a twofold increase since 1980, when there were 6.7 million people with asthma. Although a substantial increase has been noted in people between the ages of 18 and 44, the greatest increase in this country has occurred in children from infancy to four years of age, with 1 in 45 afflicted in 1980, increasing to 1 in 13 in 1998. There are some cities—for example, Philadelphia—where the incidence among children can be as high as 1 in 4. Children currently comprise about 5 million of the 17 million sufferers. Al-

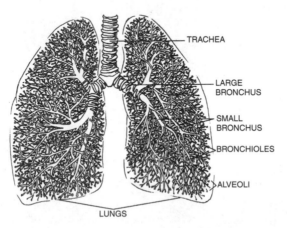

FIGURE 2.1   *The Bronchial Tree of the Lungs*

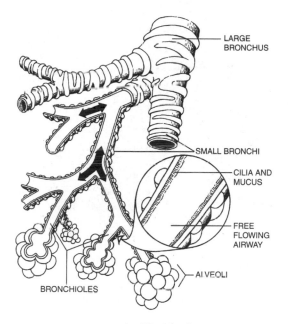

LARGE
BRONCHUS

SMALL BRONCHI

CILIA AND
MUCUS

FREE
FLOWING
AIRWAY

ALVEOLI

BRONCHIOLES

FIGURE 2.2   *Healthy Lung*

though the total incidence of asthma is 14 percent higher among black children than white, they suffer to a much greater extent with the condition. The rates of hospital admissions, emergency room visits, and deaths is dramatically higher for poor blacks and Hispanics than it is for whites. Blacks are 2.5 times more likely to die of the disease than whites. In a 1999 study performed by the Center for Children's Health and the Environment at Mount Sinai School of Medicine in New York City, it was determined that hospitalization rates were as much as 21 times higher in poorer, minority areas than in the affluent communities with the highest incidence of asthma. High rates of hospitalization are one of the most accurate indications of the widespread severity of the disease. The director of the center that performed the study, Dr. Philip Landrigan, said, "I have to suspect that other large urban areas where conditions are similar are going to find similar kinds of patterns emerge as well." This same study revealed stark differences in the hospitalization

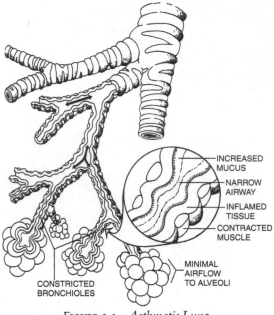

INCREASED MUCUS
NARROW AIRWAY
INFLAMED TISSUE
CONTRACTED MUSCLE
MINIMAL AIRFLOW TO ALVEOLI
CONSTRICTED BRONCHIOLES

FIGURE 2.3 *Asthmatic Lung*

rates between the poor and the richer neighborhoods for *all* age groups. The CDC has reported that the disease is most prevalent in the heavily populated areas of the Northeast, Chicago, Denver, Los Angeles, and Oakland.

Nationally, the CDC also reports that the incidence of acute asthma among children has increased 100 percent in the past decade, despite the development of medications that are highly effective if taken properly. Asthma is the leading chronic condition and the most common cause of hospitalization among American children, with about 5 million per year. Deaths among children with the condition rose by 78 percent from 1980 to 1993, and blacks between the ages of 5 and 24 are 4 to 6 times more likely to die from asthma than whites. It kills nearly 6,000 Americans annually, and as a nation we spend about $14 billion treating the disease. It is also the most common medical reason for school absence and the most frequent cause of trips to hospital emergency rooms.

RISK FACTORS AND CAUSES

The epidemic of asthma is not just an American problem—asthma prevalence is rapidly increasing in many of the industrialized countries throughout the world. In the United Kingdom the rate of asthma among children is 1 in 7, in Australia 1 in 4, and in New Zealand 1 in 3. Interestingly enough, however, while it is the poor who suffer most in the United States, the opposite is true in much of the rest of the world. Poorer, polluted eastern Germany has far fewer asthmatics than richer, cleaner western Germany. In Africa, asthma is 56 times more prevalent in rich areas of Zimbabwe than in poor areas. The lack of understanding of this phenomenon along with its rapid unexplained worldwide increase has prompted many researchers to echo the sentiments of Jeff Fredberg, a Harvard School of Public Health physiology program director who said, *"In 1999 we don't know what asthma is. It's a shocking state of affairs."* The fact is that the underlying cause of this epidemic remains one of the biggest mysteries in modern medicine.

Although it's classified as a single disease, most experts now think that asthma is a host of similar ailments, and they can't figure out how to differentiate among them. Approximately 90 percent of children (50 percent of adults) with asthma have *allergies*—to pollen, food, mold, or something else in the air or that they ingest. About 70 percent of asthmatics also have chronic *sinusitis,* which often precedes the asthma. The predicament is described by CDC epidemiologist David Mannino, who documented the dramatic rise of asthma as "a bunch of blind men on an elephant, and we're not even sure we're on an elephant." In spite of the confusion as to what's causing the epidemic, there are a number of factors that most medical scientists will agree are the most frequent triggers for an asthma attack. They include:

- Air pollutants, both indoor and outdoor (especially car exhaust—diesel is the worst)
- Pollen

- Tobacco smoke, including secondhand smoke
- Mold
- Dust mites
- Cockroach parts
- Animal dander, especially that of cats
- The common cold
- Exercise
- Occupational hazards—bakers (flour), automotive painters (isocyanates), auto and airplane mechanics, urethane workers (metals), jewelry makers (platinum salts), chemical industry workers

Several recent studies that have spawned new theories about the causes of asthma are also gaining support within the scientific community:

- Excessive cleanliness and an unchallenged immune system cause some immune cells (T helper-2 cells) to overreact to simple things in the environment, such as dust mites or mold.
- Obesity and inactivity from TV and computer games—asthmatics' and obese children's lungs don't stretch and function as normal lungs do. Most severe asthmatic children are overweight. One study showed that the children in the highest group of body mass index (BMI)—the most definitive measure for obesity—were roughly twice as likely to develop asthma as those in the lower group.
- Antibiotic use in infancy: The greater the number of courses of antibiotics during the first year of life, the greater the risk of developing asthma.
- Insufficient breast-feeding: Children who had been exclusively breast-fed for the first 4 months of life, had a substantially reduced risk of developing asthma, and if they did have asthma, their symptoms were less severe than children who received milk other than breast milk in the first 4 months of life.
- Genetics and breast milk: Breast-fed children whose mothers had asthma were almost 5 times more likely to develop asthma

compared with breast-fed children whose mothers did not have asthma.

• Elevated STAT-1: In a 1999 study, asthmatics were found to have extremely high levels of a protein called STAT 1, normally found in the cells of the mucous membrane lining the bronchioles. This protein that normally helps to defend the lungs against viruses is, in asthmatics, being excessively produced and causing inflammation of the airway *without* a virus being present. This finding may lead the way to a genetic treatment for asthma—a gene that's delivered into the airway that produces a protein that can suppress STAT-1.

Asthma, like every other chronic disease, is a complex condition with multiple risk factors and causes. Based on my clinical experience, I fully concur with each of the factors listed above, although I cannot offer an educated opinion on the "cleanliness" or STAT-1 theories. I have to admit that having practiced for almost thirty years in Denver, until very recently I was absolutely certain that the primary cause for the asthma epidemic was *air pollution*. You might have noticed that the highest-incidence areas in the United States (mentioned above) coincide with the most polluted areas, including Denver. Separate studies in New York, Connecticut, New Jersey, and Georgia from 1988 to 1990 all confirmed a strong association between the ozone levels in smog and the severity of asthma. On days when ozone levels were highest, asthma attacks increased by 25 to 30 percent. Ozone in the lower, breathable part of the atmosphere (within 1,000 feet of the earth's surface) has been repeatedly shown to be harmful to human and animal health, crops, and forests. In the upper atmosphere, the protective layer of ozone is beneficial, absorbing the harmful rays (ultraviolet B) sunlight. A Canadian study in 1991 suggested that ozone can increase the lungs' responsiveness to allergens, such as ragweed or grass. Based on that research, it was recommended that during periods of high ozone, asthmatics should be inactive, stay inside, and use air conditioners. The other outdoor air pollutants—particulates (especially diesel exhaust), hydrocarbons, nitrogen dioxide, and sulfur dioxide—have all been scientifically proven to be harmful to the respiratory tract. In fact, the EPA believes that air pollution is *killing* over 60,000 Americans every year. Another piece of circumstantial evidence supporting this theory is that most epidemiologists date the onset for the dramatic rise in asthma to around 1980. I first became convinced of the air pollution/respiratory disease link in 1981, when the National Center for Health Statistics, a division of the CDC, for the first time ranked sinusitis as America's most common chronic disease. It has continued to increase and has remained in that position ever since. Asthma is currently ranked as the eighth most common condition, while allergies are fourth. This means that there are over 90 million Americans, more than 1 out of every 3 people, who suffer with a chronic respiratory condition. In the late 1960s not one of these three respiratory ailments was among the top ten. It seems blatantly clear that the sea of toxic pollutants in which we are immersed and inhale on average 23,000 times a day is assaulting our body's air filter—the nose and sinuses—and rapidly destroying our entire respiratory tract. Indoor air pollution is far more insidious and potentially more devastating than outdoor air, since we spend over 90 percent of our time indoors. The entire list of indoor pollutants follows in Table 2.1, but those that have the greatest adverse effect on asthmatics are: secondhand smoke, house dust, mold, dust mites, animal dander, and cockroach parts.

During the past two years, however, my thinking has changed and I have greatly expanded my perspective on the causes of asthma. I still believe that air pollution is a major contributor, but I am now equally convinced that there is a profound immune dysfunction in asthmatics. This change has resulted from the Mayo Clinic study implicating fungus as a primary cause of sinusitis; the study demonstrating the effectiveness of Diflucan (an antifungal medication) in treating asthmatics (refer to page 121); my own Sinus Survival study, in which Diflucan was highly effective in treating chronic sinusitis as well as asthma (three of the patients in the study also had asthma, which improved significantly along with their sinusitis); the proliferation

Table 2.1
Indoor Air Pollutants

Automotive Fumes
Sources include outdoor traffic, outdoor parking lots, and outdoor
loading and unloading spaces, as well as indoor garages.

Chemicals and Chemical Solutions (Chemicals that affect indoor air
quality are those associated with architecture, the interior, artifacts,
and maintenance.)
Fungicides and pesticides in carpet-cleaning residues and sprays;
formaldehyde, used in the manufacture of insulation, plywood,
fiberboard, furniture, and wood paneling; toxic solvents in oil-
based paints, finishes, and wall sealants; aerosol sprays; office
equipment chemicals, especially photocopiers and computers

Combustion Products
Tobacco smoke*
Coal- or wood-burning fireplaces and stoves
Fuel combustion gases from gas-fired appliances such as ranges,
clothes dryers, water heaters, and fireplaces. (They produce nitrogen dioxide, carbon monoxide, nitrous oxides, sulfur oxides, hydrocarbons, and formaldehyde.)

Ion Depletion or Imbalance
Too few negative ions
Excess of positive ions over negative ions

Microorganisms (primarily from humidifiers, air conditioners, and
any other building components affected by excessive moisture)
Bacteria
Viruses
Molds
Dust mites (usually found in carpets in more humid areas)
Cockroaches

Particulates
Dust
Pollen
Animal dander
Particles (frayed materials)
Asbestos

Radionuclides

Radon, a radioactive gas emitted from the earth that enters homes
   primarily through basements, crawl spaces, and water supply, especially from wells. (It can attach to the particulates of cigarette
   smoke, dust particles, and natural aerosols.)

*From all of the available scientific data, tobacco smoke is the most unhealthy
indoor air pollutant.

of resistant bacteria resulting from the overuse of antibiotics;
several new Functional Lab Tests that have shed new light on the
possible causes of asthma (see below); and my two-week trip to
New Zealand during the summer of 2000. I was invited to introduce holistic medicine to a populace with the second-highest
incidence of asthma in the world and no definitive explanation
for this phenomenon. And there is almost *no air pollution* in New
Zealand. However, their proximity to the South Pole and the
expanding hole in our protective ozone layer gave me a clue. I
remembered that there have been a few studies linking the increased exposure to the ultraviolet light resulting from the thinning ozone layer to a *weakened immune response.* This ominous
environmental catastrophe-in-the-making is probably already
impacting both New Zealand and Australia to a greater extent
than almost any other country. Although these two countries already have among the highest incidence in the world of both
asthma and skin cancer, the rest of us are not far behind. We are
all feeling the impact of this global disaster resulting from our
unconscious and wanton destruction of our atmosphere. The
pollutants themselves have been directly responsible for helping
to destroy our respiratory tracts and to increase our risk of developing most forms of cancer. Now indirectly, by creating a
hole in our protective shield, they are causing dysfunction in our
immune system. I have said this many times before, but never
more strongly than this: *"As we continue to devastate our environment, we are in the process of destroying our species."* I strongly believe that the combination of breathing highly polluted air and
their subsequent irritation and inflammation of the mucosa lin-

ing the entire respiratory tract, along with the gradual weakening of our immunity, is the primary cause of the respiratory disease epidemic—asthma, sinusitis, and allergies. That lethal combination is probably to some extent responsible for far more than just respiratory disease. It may be a few years before scientists can prove it, but there has to be some explanation for the proliferation of physical disorders related to an impaired immune system during the past two decades. These diseases, which were unknown or quite rare as recently as twenty years ago, are now turning into epidemics. The Epstein-Barr virus, the cause of mononucleosis, is now in part responsible for chronic fatigue syndrome and fibromyalgia. Besides the lung conditions (asthma, chronic bronchitis, emphysema, and lung cancer), herpes simplex infections, candidiasis, "ecologic illness (or multiple chemical sensitivity)," lupus (systemic lupus erythematosus), multiple sclerosis, ALS (amyotrophic lateral sclerosis), and AIDS (acquired immunodeficiency syndrome) are all examples of this phenomenon.

Holistic medicine is focused on treating the underlying *causes,* or dysfunctional patterns of physiology and behavior, of chronic illness. If we can determine a cause, or interacting multiple causes, we can more accurately make therapeutic choices that can potentially effect a cure while also improving quality and longevity of life. Traditionally, allopathic medicine's (as practiced by most M.D.s) sole focus is diagnosing, or naming, the disease, and then addressing the management of symptoms. As you'll see in the following pages of this chapter, that is certainly the case with the treatment of asthma. But this is an end-point approach, with the outcomes for chronic illness being very limited (the usual outcome is "learning to live with your illness"). Allopathic medicine may save your life, but it often does not uncover, mitigate, or eliminate the multiple causes of chronic disease. And more important, conventional therapy will usually not have a significant impact on long-term improvement of function.

Lab tests have come very far in the last several years in helping to determine underlying causes and dysfunctions that aren't necessarily a disease or pathology. These new tests, called functional lab tests, are designed to go beyond traditional testing and accurately measure underlying causal factors that may be a critical factor in perpetuating your symptoms. A number of labs across the country now do functional testing, which provides both the practitioner and the patient with much more useful information for determining the unique biochemical causes and factors impacting your health.

Below is a brief list of those functional lab tests that Dr. Nelson and I believe are most important for evaluating and determining the best course of personalized treatment for asthma. Not only can these tests help to clarify the specific dysfunction that may be contributing to your asthma, they can also help to determine if the treatment is working since they can provide objective markers to demonstrate improvement. (If you choose to start the Asthma Survival Program by doing these tests with your doctor, then you should postpone beginning the Quick Fix program in Chapter 1 until after the appropriate tests have been performed and sent to the lab. See Resource Guide, page 321, for laboratories.)

1. **Comprehensive Digestive Stool Analysis with Ova and Parasites × 3.** This is probably the most comprehensive stool test in the United States. It is a three-day collection you can do at home. It is vital to determine if you have underlying dysfunction in digestion that can affect and increase toxicity in your body and prevent you from absorbing nutrients. It will reveal if you have a candida yeast infection (an increasingly significant cause of asthma) very accurately. It will also show if your gut is dysbiotic (an imbalance of the normal bacterial flora), if you might have a leaky gut (increased permeability of the intestinal lining), or if there are low-grade bacterial or parasitic infections. (Great Smokies Lab)

2. **Adrenal Stress Index Test.** This is a saliva collection test that can be done at home. This test determines your general adrenal function, by measuring tissue levels of cortisol

and DHEA. Most asthmatics have low adrenal function, which affects allergies, breathing, and energy. They also do a salivary secretory IgA, which shows how well your front-line mucus immunity is functioning. It is usually low in asthmatics because it is depleted in the face of infections, allergies, and medications. Anti-Gliadin SigA is tested to determine allergy to gluten in the diet. (Diagnos-tech)

3. **Food Allergy Testing.** Numerous labs offer IgE and IgG Rast testing to determine immediate and delayed-onset allergies. (Great Smokies is a good lab for this test.)

4. **Functional Liver Detoxification panel.** This is a liver challenge test to determine how well the liver is detoxifying. When you are taking medications, are experiencing allergies or recurrent infections, are not eating well, and are under stress, the liver slows down its ability to detoxify and increases free-radical production, which ultimately damages immunity. This simple, inexpensive test can help determine the appropriate antioxidant and detoxification program for your treatment. (Great Smokies Lab)

5. **Intestinal Permeability.** This is another test you can easily do at home. You are determining if your intestinal lining is "leaky" and allowing large, undigested molecules to be absorbed, which can then trigger allergic and asthmatic responses. You challenge your gut with a drink made from simple sugars, lactulose and mannitol. If high levels show up in urine or saliva, then you have a leaky gut and must take nutritional steps to heal it. (Great Smokies Lab)

6. **RBC Magnesium.** This is a much more accurate test to determine magnesium levels than are regular blood serum tests. The blood serum may be normal, yet you may not be absorbing adequate amounts of magnesium into your cells. Adequate magnesium levels in tissue are critical for an asthma patient, as you will learn in Chapter 4. (Most labs can perform this test.)

In summary, the Asthma Survival Program is based on the belief that asthma is primarily caused by:

1. Air pollution—both outdoor (ozone, particulates [esp. diesel], nitrogen and sulfur dioxide, hydrocarbons) and indoor pollutants.
2. Immune dysfunction, secondary to:
   a. Overuse of antibiotics and prednisone—contributing to immune suppression, antibiotic-resistant bacteria, and infections and bowel dysfunction caused by fungal and candida albicans organisms.
   b. Emotional stress:
      • grief—the physical and/or emotional loss of a parent (usually father)
      • enmeshment, a smothering love, between parent (usually mother) and child
      • lack of bonding between parents and child; specifically, a lack of physical affection
      • lack of bonding between parents of an asthmatic child
   c. Allergies and sensitivities to both food and airborne particles:
      • most common foods—milk and dairy, wheat or any gluten grain, egg, peanut, soy, chocolate, cocoa, corn, citrus, fish (cold-water fish are usually OK—salmon, tuna), shellfish, yeast, onion, garlic; aspirin, food preservatives and additives (sulfites especially, MSG, tartrazine or yellow dyes, sodium benzoate)
   d. Thinning ozone layer

CONVENTIONAL MEDICAL TREATMENT

I recognize that this will be the section of the book with which the majority of you are most familiar, since you have probably been working with a physician to treat your asthma. Therefore, my intent is simply to add to your understanding of the conventional approach, to help you appreciate to a greater extent why you've been prescribed the medications that you're taking, and to assist you in more effectively preventing asthma attacks from occurring. This information will also help you to begin incorporating the Asthma Survival Program as a complement to what you are presently doing.

According to the 1997 version of *Guidelines for the Diagnosis and Management of Asthma,* issued by the National Heart, Lung, and Blood Institute (NHLBI) of the National Institutes of Health (NIH), effective management of asthma has the following *goals:*

- To prevent and control chronic and troublesome symptoms (e.g., coughing or breathlessness in the night, in the early morning, or after exertion)
- To maintain near-normal pulmonary function rates
- To maintain normal activity levels, including exercise
- To prevent acute episodes of asthma requiring emergency room visits and hospitalizations
- To avoid adverse effects of asthma medications
- To attain a level of asthma care that is satisfactory to patients and families

Effective *management* of asthma relies on four integral components:

- Objective measures of lung function, not only to assess but also to monitor each patient's asthma
- Pharmacologic therapy
- Environmental measures to control allergens and irritants
- Patient education

Although patient education, environmental measures, and pulmonary function tests are all an integral part of the treatment program, the attainment of these goals for managing chronic asthma relies heavily on the proper administration of pharmaceutical drugs. The treatment of an acute asthma attack, often considered a medical emergency, is totally dependent on medication. Conventional medicine frequently performs "miracles" for these patients, who are unable to breathe and are confronting death by suffocation. In these critical situations, the conventional approach is clearly superior to anything else.

Notice, however, that the objective in treating chronic asthma is "management." There is no mention of *curing* this disease. Conventional medical belief is that asthma *cannot* be cured but that asthma symptoms can be controlled. The general *principles involved in managing chronic asthma* include:

- Treat the underlying pathology of asthma. First-line therapy should focus on preventing or reversing the airway inflammation that is a principal factor in the airway hyperresponsiveness that characterizes asthma and determines symptoms, disease severity, and possibly mortality. (In recent years, researchers have implicated leukotrienes as the primary cause of the inflammation of asthma. Leukotrienes are a group of chemical compounds released by white blood cells—leukocytes—that can also cause the mucous membrane to swell, the airway muscles to constrict, and increased mucus to be secreted. It is due to the discovery of leukotrienes that anti-inflammatory medications have become a key component of asthma treatment regimens. But what is it that triggers the release of the leukotrienes to begin the cycle of events resulting in wheezing?)
- Tailor general therapy guidelines to individual needs. Specific asthma therapy, dictated by the severity of the disease, medication tolerance, and sensitivity to environmental allergens, must be selected to fit the needs of individual patients.
- Treat asthma triggers, associated conditions, and special problems: Exposure to known allergens and irritants must be reduced or eliminated; colds, sinus infections, middle-ear infections (otitis media), and allergic rhinitis can set off or aggravate asthma. Treatment of a known trigger prior to exposure, such as exercise, is recommended. Influenza vaccinations and pneumococcal vaccines should be considered for patients with moderate or severe asthma.
- Seek consultation with an asthma specialist for pulmonary

function studies, evaluation of the role of allergy and irritants, or evaluation of the medication plan if the goals of therapy are not achieved.

- Use step-care pharmacologic therapy. An aim of this therapy is to use the optimum medication needed to maintain control with minimal risk for adverse effects. The step-care approach, in which the number of medications and frequency of administration are increased as necessary, is used to achieve this aim.

- Monitor continually. Continual monitoring, including pulmonary function tests and regular visits to your physician, are necessary to assure that therapeutic goals are met. The consistent use of a *peak flow meter* is an integral component of your asthma management and should become a skill that you develop with minimal coaching from your physician. It is a handheld device that is relatively simple to use and is inexpensive. This meter measures how fast you can expel (breathe out) air from your lungs. The recorded measurement then gives you an idea of how well your lungs are working, and is able to warn you of an upcoming asthma attack even before you notice any increase of symptoms on your own. This early warning gives you the chance to take medication to stop the attack before it becomes a crisis. The peak flow meter can also be quite helpful in identifying triggers for attacks, in modifying dosages of medications, and in monitoring your progress as you gradually implement the Asthma Survival Program. The results can be recorded on the Symptom Chart (page 62).

Asthma Medications

In the 1997 NHLBI Guidelines, asthma drugs have been reclassified as *quick-relief* medications and medications used for *long-term control*. All of the medications in both groups are either anti-inflammatory agents or bronchodilators. The anti-inflammatories interrupt the development of bronchial inflammation and have a preventive action. They also mitigate ongoing inflammatory reactions in the airways. The *anti-inflammatory drugs* include:

- Oral corticosteroids, such as prednisone, prednisolone, or methylprednisolone; these can be used for both short-acting quick relief and/or long-term control
- Inhaled corticosteroids, such as beclomethasone (Beclovent, Vanceril), triamcinolone (Azmacort), flunisolide (AeroBid), or fluticasone (Flovent); these are all used for long-term control
- Cromolyn sodium (Intal) or cromolyn-like compounds, such as nedocromil sodium (Tilade), for long-term control
- Leukotriene modifiers, such as zafirlukast (Accolate, Singulair) and zileuton (Zyflo). These antileukotrienes are the first new class of asthma medications in over twenty years. Although they have anti-inflammatory properties, they are less potent than corticosteroids. They are currently approved for use for long-term control in adults and in children over 12, and work by interfering with key mediators in asthma, cysteinyl leukotrienes.

The *bronchodilators* act principally to dilate the airways by relaxing bronchial smooth muscle. They include beta-adrenergic agonists, methylxanthines, and anticholinergics. Inhaled beta-2 agonists are the medication of choice for treatment of acute asthma attacks and for the prevention of exercise-induced asthma. They are best administered via metered dose inhaler or nebulizer. Although they have also been used for long-term control of persistent moderate-to-severe asthma, studies suggest that prolonged, regular administration (as opposed to as-needed use) of a potent beta-agonist might result in diminished control of asthma and might even be a contributing factor in the increasing death toll in asthmatic children. As a result, there are currently beta agonists that are used strictly for long-term control. The most often prescribed bronchodilators include:

- Short-acting beta-2 agonists, such as albuterol (Proventil), bitolterol (Tornalate), pirbuterol (Maxair), and terbutaline (Brethaire)

- Long-acting beta-2 agonists, such as sustained-release albuterol (Proventil Repetabs), and salmetereol (Serevent)
- The methylxanthine theophylline, which is used for long-term control in either elixir, syrup, or timed-release tablets and capsules

There are a number of new asthma drugs that are currently being studied and some that will soon be available for use. Most are in the anti-inflammatory category and will probably reduce the need for the daily use of corticosteroid inhalers in long-term treatment. One new medication, Advair Diskus, is an inhaler that combines a long-acting bronchodilator with a corticosteroid, making it a bit more convenient to treat this condition.

NHLBI Classification of Asthma Severity and Pharmacological Treatment

Step 1: Mild Intermittent Asthma
- Symptoms no more than twice a week
- Nighttime symptoms not more than twice a week
- Lung function: FEV-1 (forced expiratory volume in 1 second = the amount of air you can forcibly blow out of your lungs in 1 second) or PEF (peak expiratory flow) 80 percent or more of predicted value and varies by less than 20 percent.
- Flare-ups are brief (from a few hours to a few days), with varying intensity.
- Asymptomatic, with normal PEF between asthma flare-ups

TREATMENT
Short-Term Control: Inhaled, short-acting beta-2 agonist as needed for symptoms. The use of short-acting, inhaled beta 2 agonist more than two times per week may indicate the need to initiate long-term control therapy.
Long-Term Control: No daily medication needed.

Step 2: Mild Persistent Asthma
- Symptoms more than twice a week but less than once a day
- Nighttime symptoms more than twice a month
- FEV-1 or PEF 80 percent or more of predicted value, and the PEF varies by 20 to 30 percent
- Flare-ups may affect activity

TREATMENT

Short-Term Control: Short-acting, inhaled beta-2 agonist as needed for symptoms. *Note:* Using short-acting, inhaled beta-2 agonist on a daily basis or an increase in frequency of use indicates the need for additional long-term control therapy.

Long-Term Control:

One daily medication needed: Inhaled low-dose corticosteroids; *or* cromolyn or nedocromil (children usually begin with a trial of cromolyn or neocromil)

Alternative therapies, but not preferred: Sustained-release theophylline to serum concentration 5 to 15 mcg/ml; *or* zafirlukast or zileuton (leukotriene modifiers) may be considered in patients older than 11 years of age.

Step 3: Moderate Persistent Asthma
- Daily symptoms
- Daily use of inhaled, short-acting beta-2 agonist
- Nighttime symptoms more than once a week
- Flare-ups affect activity.
- Flare-up two or more times a week; may last for days
- FEV-1 or PEF between 60 and 80 percent of predicted value, and PEF varies by more than 30 percent

TREATMENT

Short-Term Control: Short-acting, inhaled beta-2 agonist as needed for symptoms. *Note:* Using short-acting beta-2 agonist on a daily basis or an increase in frequency of use indicates the need for additional long-term control.

Long-Term Control:

Daily medication: Inhaled corticosteroid (medium dose); *or* inhaled corticosteroid (low-medium dose); *and* long-acting, inhaled beta-2 agonist, sustained-release theophylline, or long-acting beta-2 agonist tablets. *If needed,* inhaled corticosteroid (medium-high dose); *and* long-acting, inhaled beta-2 agonist, sustained-release theophylline, or long-acting beta-2 agonist tablets.

Step 4: Severe Persistent Asthma
- Continual symptoms
- Limited physical activity
- Frequent nighttime symptoms
- Frequent flare-ups
- FEV-1 or PEF less than 60 percent of predicted value, and PEF varies by more than 30 percent

TREATMENT

Short-Term Control: Short-acting, inhaled beta-2 agonist as needed for symptoms.

   Note: Using short-acting beta-2 agonist on a daily basis or an increase in frequency of use indicates the need for additional long-term control.

Long-Term Control:

Daily Medication: Inhaled corticosteroid (high dose); *and* long-acting inhaled beta-2 agonist, sustained-release theophylline, or long-acting beta-2 agonist tablets; *and* corticosteroid tablets *or* syrup.

To gain control of moderate and severe asthma, it is recommended that therapy be initiated with moderate to high-dose inhaled or even oral corticosteroids. Once control is achieved, the treatment should be rapidly reduced to the level required to maintain control.

Patient Education

With each stage of the Step Therapy of Asthma, patient education is an essential component. It allows the patient to participate in their own management of the condition and increases their adherence to the treatment program. The key elements of the educational program are:

1. Basic facts about asthma, including the importance of inflammation
2. The role of medication and the importance of long-term control
3. Skills—the use of inhalers; how to monitor symptoms and use peak of the peak flow meter
4. Environmental control measures
5. When and how to take action measures—physicians are urged to provide patients with two written treatment plans, one describing daily self-management and one for managing acute flare-ups at home

Although the above classification and the step therapy treatment guidelines have been widely accepted by the vast majority of asthma specialists (mainly allergists or pulmonologists), *compliance* with these guidelines by both physicians and patients is actually quite low. Even though adherence to step therapy is better among patients of specialists than it is for those treated by primary care physicians, compliance studies have revealed surprisingly low rates of daily use of preventive long-term control medication and especially the peak flow meter. As a result, many patients are not meeting the goals of asthma therapy as listed on page 39, and numerous unnecessary hospitalizations, emergency room visits, and deaths have occurred. One of the greatest problems in the management of asthma is the sheer inconvenience of juggling multiple inhalers and other medications. Worldwide sales of asthma drugs are currently in excess of $7 billion and are expected to increase to more than $12 billion by 2003. According to industry analysts, "Any new treatment that eliminates the need for multiple inhalers could easily reap more than $2 billion annually." In the chapters that follow, you'll find such a treatment. However, rather than a drug company, you will reap all of the rewards. In spite of the fact that asthma is a potentially life-threatening condition and an asthma attack can be a terrifying experience, most people in our society remain crisis-oriented and act only when they're unable to breathe. Only a small percentage are willing to take responsibility for their care and practice preventive medicine. However, to fully benefit from the Asthma Survival Program (a powerful preventive approach), you must be willing to become an active participant in your own treatment. Regularly monitoring your symptoms, daily use of preventive medication (if you have mild, moderate, or severe persistent asthma), and the use of the peak flow meter are all essential to your success with this holistic medical program. But they comprise only a small portion of the daily practices I'm recommending. I cannot emphasize enough the value of a strong *commitment.* If you are willing to commit to the full-time job of healing your life—learning to care for, nurture, and love your lungs, your body, your mind, and your spirit—then you will breathe freely and move well beyond the management of asthma to the experience of being fully alive.

Chapter 3

HOLISTIC HEALTH: THE THRIVING SELF-TEST

"The only thing I know that truly heals people is unconditional love."

ELISABETH KÜBLER-ROSS, M.D.

M ost people who read this book have asthma, and possibly sinus and allergy problems, and don't consider themselves to be particularly healthy. But **what is health?** The conditioning that the majority of us have grown up with has taught us to define health as the absence of illness. We may respond to the question "Are you healthy?" by thinking, *I'm not sick, so I must be healthy.* Yet the words *health, heal,* and *holy* are all derived from the same Old English word, *haelan,* which means **to make whole.** Viewed from this perspective, two questions that more directly and accurately address the issue of health are "Do you love your life?" and "Are you happy to be alive?" Health is far more than simply a matter of not feeling ill: It is the daily experience of *wholeness and balance—a state of being fully alive in body, mind, and spirit.* Such a condition could also be called optimal health, or holistic health, or wellness. I call it *thriving.* Helping you to achieve this state of total well-being is the primary objective of this book. *As a by-product of that enlivening process, your lungs will heal and your asthma will either improve significantly or be cured.*

HALLMARKS OF OPTIMAL HEALTH

Optimal health results from harmony and balance in the physical, environmental, mental, emotional, spiritual, and social aspects of our lives. When this harmonious balance is present, we experience the *unlimited and unimpeded free flow of life-force energy throughout our body, mind, and spirit.* Around the world, this energy is known by many names. The Chinese call it *qi* ("chee"), the Japanese refer to it as *ki,* in India it is known as *prana,* and in Hebrew it is *chai.* But in the Western world, the phrase that comes closest to capturing the feeling generated by this energy is *unconditional love,* regarded by holistic physicians as *our most powerful healer.*

Although each of us has the capacity to nurture and to heal ourselves, most of us have yet to tap into this wellspring of loving life energy. Yet there is no one who can better administer this life-enhancing elixir to you than you yourself.

By committing to caring for yourself in the manner recommended in the following chapters, you will in essence be learning how to better *give and receive love*—to yourself and others. As a result, you will be enhancing the flow of life-force energy throughout every aspect of your life. This holistic healing process will also provide you with the opportunity to safely and effectively treat your asthma and any other physical, mental, and spiritual conditions that may be impeding the flow of healing energy in your life.

Living a holistically healthy lifestyle can facilitate the realization of your ideal life vision in accordance with both your personal and professional goals. But since the majority of us are aware of health only as a condition of not being sick, a mental image of what living holistically means is needed in order to achieve it. Briefly, let's examine this state of optimal well-being to give you a glimpse of what it looks and feels like.

A list of the six components of health follows, the first italicized item in each category encompassing the essence of that component. For example, physical health can be simply described as a condition of *high energy and vitality,* while mental health is a state of *peace of mind and contentment*. The italicized items also serve as a health gauge you can use to measure your progress in each area.

PHYSICAL HEALTH
High energy and vitality
- Freedom from, or high adaptability to, pain, dysfunction, and disability
- A strong immune system
- A body that feels light, balanced, strong, flexible, and has good aerobic capacity
- Ability to meet physical challenges and perform exceptionally
- Full capacity of all five senses and a healthy libido

ENVIRONMENTAL HEALTH
Harmony with your environment (neither harming nor being harmed)
- Awareness of your connectedness with nature
- Feeling grounded—comfort and security within your surroundings
- Respect and appreciation for your home, the Earth, and all of her inhabitants
- Contact with the earth; breathing healthy air; drinking pure water; eating uncontaminated food; exposure to the sun, fire, or candlelight; immersion in warm water (all on a daily basis)

MENTAL HEALTH
Peace of mind and contentment
- A job that you love doing
- Optimism
- A sense of humor
- Financial well-being
- Living your life vision
- The ability to express your creativity and talents
- The capacity to make healthy decisions

EMOTIONAL HEALTH

Self-acceptance and high self-esteem
- The capacity to identify, express, experience, and accept all of your feelings, both painful and joyful
- Awareness of the intimate connection between your physical and emotional bodies
- The ability to confront your greatest fears
- The fulfillment of your capacity to play
- Peak experiences on a regular basis

SPIRITUAL HEALTH

Experience of unconditional love / absence of fear
- Soul awareness and a personal relationship with God or Spirit
- Trust in your intuition and an openness to change
- Gratitude
- Creating a sacred space on a regular basis through prayer, meditation, walking in nature, observing a Sabbath day, or other rituals
- Sense of purpose
- Being present in every moment

SOCIAL HEALTH

Intimacy with a spouse or partner, relative, or close friend
- Effective communication
- Forgiveness
- Sense of belonging to a support group or community
- Touch and/or physical intimacy on a daily basis
- Selflessness and altruism

The Thriving Self-Test

Now that you understand the six categories that constitute optimal health, it's time to measure how close you are to *thriving* in each area. The following questionnaire is designed to provide you with a much clearer idea of the status of your health in all six areas. You can use the results of the test to guide you through the rest of the book and it can become a blueprint for restructuring your life. You can also measure your progress by retaking the test every two or three months.

Answer the questions in each section below and total your score. Each response will be a number from 0 to 5. Please refer to the frequency described within the parentheses (e.g., "2 to 3 times/week") when answering questions about an *activity*—for example, "Do you maintain a healthy diet?" However, when the question refers to an *attitude* or an *emotion* (most of the Mind and Spirit questions—for example, "Do you have a sense of humor?"), the response is more subjective and less exact, and you should refer to the terms describing the frequency, such as *often* or *daily*, but not to the numbered frequencies in parentheses.

0 = Never or almost never (once a year or less)
1 = Seldom (2 to 12 times/year)
2 = Occasionally (2 to 4 times/month)
3 = Often (2 to 3 times/week)
4 = Regularly (4 to 6 times/week)
5 = Daily (every day)

BODY: PHYSICAL AND ENVIRONMENTAL HEALTH

_____ 1. Do you maintain a healthy diet (low fat, low sugar, fresh fruits, grains, and vegetables)?

_____ 2. Is your daily water intake adequate (at least ½ oz./lb of body weight; 160 lbs. = 80 ounces)?

_____ 3. Are you within 20 percent of your ideal body weight?

_____ 4. Do you feel physically attractive?

_____ 5. Do you fall asleep easily and sleep soundly?

_____ 6. Do you awaken in the morning feeling well rested?

_____ 7. Do you have more than enough energy to meet your daily responsibilities?

_____ 8. Are your five senses acute?

_____ 9. Do you take time to experience sensual pleasure?

_____ 10. Do you schedule regular massage or deep-tissue body work?

_____ 11. Does your sexual relationship feel gratifying?

_____ 12. Do you engage in regular physical workouts (lasting at least 20 minutes)?

_____ 13. Do you have good endurance or aerobic capacity?

_____ 14. Do you breathe abdominally for at least a few minutes?

_____ 15. Do you maintain physically challenging goals?

_____ 16. Are you physically strong?

_____ 17. Do you do some stretching exercises?

_____ 18. Are you free of chronic aches, pains, ailments, and diseases?

_____ 19. Do you have regular effortless bowel movements?

_____ 20. Do you understand the causes of your chronic physical problems?

_____ 21. Are you free of any drug (including caffeine and nicotine) or alcohol dependency?

_____ 22. Do you live and work in a healthy environment with respect to clean air, water, and indoor pollution?

_____ 23. Do you feel energized or empowered by nature?

_____ 24. Do you feel a strong connection with and appreciation for your body, your home, and your environment?

_____ 25. Do you have an awareness of life-force energy, or *qi* ("chee")?

_____   TOTAL BODY SCORE

MIND: MENTAL AND EMOTIONAL HEALTH

_____ 1. Do you have specific goals in your personal and professional life?

_____ 2. Do you have the ability to concentrate for extended periods of time?

_____ 3. Do you use visualization or mental imagery to help you attain your goals or enhance your performance?

_____ 4. Do you believe it is possible to change?

_____ 5. Can you meet your financial needs and desires?

_____ 6. Is your outlook basically optimistic?

_____ 7. Do you give yourself more supportive messages than critical messages?

_____ 8. Does your job utilize all of your greatest talents?

_____ 9. Is your job enjoyable and fulfilling?

_____ 10. Are you willing to take risks or make mistakes in order to succeed?

_____ 11. Are you able to adjust beliefs and attitudes as a result of learning from painful experiences?

_____ 12. Do you have a sense of humor?

_____ 13. Do you maintain peace of mind and tranquillity?

_____ 14. Are you free from a strong need for control or the need to be right?

_____ 15. Are you able to fully experience (feel) your painful feelings such as fear, anger, sadness, and hopelessness?

_____ 16. Are you aware of and able to safely express fear?

_____ 17. Are you aware of and able to safely express anger?

_____ 18. Are you aware of and able to safely express sadness (or cry)?

_____ 19. Are you accepting of all your feelings?

_____ 20. Do you engage in meditation, contemplation, or psycho-therapy to better understand your feelings?

_____ 21. Is your sleep free from disturbing dreams?

_____ 22. Do you explore the symbolism and emotional content of your dreams?

_____ 23. Do you take the time to relax, or make time for activities that constitute the abandon or absorption of play?

_____ 24. Do you experience feelings of exhilaration?

_____ 25. Do you enjoy high self-esteem?

_____ TOTAL MIND SCORE

SPIRIT: SPIRIT AND SOCIAL HEALTH

_____ 1. Do you actively commit time to your spiritual life?

_____ 2. Do you take time for prayer, meditation, or reflection?

_____ 3. Do you listen to and act upon your intuition?

_____ 4. Are creative activities a part of your work or leisure time?

_____ 5. Do you take risks?

_____ 6. Do you have faith in a God, spirit guides, or angels?

_____ 7. Are you free from anger toward God?

_____ 8. Are you grateful for the blessings in your life?

_____ 9. Do you take walks, garden, or have contact with nature?

_____ 10. Are you able to let go of your attachment to specific out-comes and embrace uncertainty?

_____ 11. Do you observe a day of rest completely away from work, dedicated to nurturing yourself and your family?

_____ 12. Can you let go of self-interest in deciding the best course of action for a given situation?

_____ 13. Do you feel a sense of purpose?

_____ 14. Do you make time to connect with young children, either your own or someone else's?

_____ 15. Are playfulness and humor important to you in your daily life?

_____ 16. Do you have the ability to forgive yourself and others?

_____ 17. Have you demonstrated the willingness to commit to a marriage or comparable long-term relationship?

_____ 18. Do you experience intimacy, besides sex, in your committed relationships?

_____ 19. Do you confide in or speak openly with one or more close friends?

_____ 20. Do you or did you feel close to your parents?

_____ 21. If you have experienced the loss of a loved one, have you fully grieved that loss?

_____ 22. Has your experience of pain enabled you to grow spiritually?

_____ 23. Do you go out of your way or give your time to help others?

_____ 24. Do you feel a sense of belonging to a group or community?

_____ 25. Do you experience unconditional love?

_____ TOTAL SPIRIT SCORE

_____ TOTAL BODY, MIND, SPIRIT SCORE

HEALTH SCALE:

325–375	Optimal Health: **THRIVING**
275–324	Excellent Health
225–274	Good Health
175–224	Fair Health
125–174	Below-Average Health
75–124	Poor Health
Less than 75	Extremely Unhealthy: **SURVIVING**

Once you complete this questionnaire, pay attention to which categories you need to make the most improvements in, and remember that *there are multiple factors that have combined to cause your asthma.* Then start to implement the tools and suggestions that are outlined in Chapters 4, 5, and 6. Chapter 4 gives you a blueprint for improving your physical and environmental health while also specifically addressing asthma, focusing on healing your mucous membranes and strengthening your immune system. Chapter 5 outlines a holistic approach for mental and emotional health, while Chapter 6 will help you enhance your spiritual and social health. Begin where you are most comfortable and take your time. You are committing to a life-changing process, one that requires patience and discipline, so proceed at your own pace. Remember, too, that everyone is unique and no two of us will follow the exact same healing path. While the science of holistic medicine provides a universal foundation and structure, its *art* lies in the writing of your own personal prescription for optimal health, so feel free to adapt the techniques in the pages ahead to tailor-make the holistic self-care program that is most ideally suited for you. Your heart will be your primary guide on this odyssey of realizing your full potential as a human being.

During the fifteen years that I've been actively engaged in this healing process, I've identified several practices that have had the deepest impact on my health, have had the most transformative effect upon my life, and will provide the greatest therapeutic benefits for your asthma. I call them the *essential 8 for optimal health:*

- Air and Breathing
- Water, Moisture, and Nasal Hygiene
- Food and Supplements
- Exercise and Rest
- Play/Passion and Meaning/Purpose
- Gratitude and Prayer
- Intimacy
- Forgiveness

As you read the following chapters and begin incorporating the Asthma Survival Program into your life, keep these *essential 8* in mind. (I've numbered them throughout the book, 1 through 8, to help you remember.) They are the basis of this holistic treatment program and can become the structure upon which the rest of your life is built.

Chapter 4

HEALING YOUR BODY
The Physical and Environmental Health Components
of the Asthma Survival Program

I f you would rather not learn to live with or prefer to do more than simply manage your asthma, then I would like to take you on a healing journey into an exciting new (yet ancient) frontier of medicine. For the past fourteen years, I have been practicing **holistic medicine** while treating asthma, sinusitis, arthritis, backache, headache, and a variety of other so-called chronic or incurable conditions. The Asthma Survival Program has its foundation in the holistic practice of treating, preventing, and potentially curing any chronic condition, as well as creating a state of optimal well-being. Although the bulk of the holistic approach is similar for any chronic condition or disease, this and the following chapters include specific dietary, nutritional supplement, and herbal recommendations; professional care therapies; and emotional factors that relate directly to treating the causes and symptoms of asthma. *Commitment* to this approach usually results in at least a significant improvement, and in many cases a cure of asthma. However, almost everyone has experienced a greater sense of well-being. This success stems primarily from the basic health orientation of the holistic approach.

Rather than focusing on the disease and just treating its symptoms—they are certainly not ignored, just perceived differently—holistic medicine addresses *causes* while restoring balance and harmony to the *whole person*. It goes far beyond the "quick fix" outlined in Chapter 1, or the repair of a "broken part," to an understanding of what can be learned from your physical dysfunction and how to use that knowledge to change your life and be free of asthma.

I was led to the practice of holistic medicine and a condition of optimal health by my painful sinuses. My guide on this healing path was, and still is, Hippocrates, who recognized 2,500 years ago the most direct and effective method for training to become a healer: "Physician, heal thyself." In the remainder of this book, Todd Nelson and I would like to guide you on a similar path, leading not only to the healing of your reactive airway disease and any other dis-ease, but to a state of holistic health. By taking the Thriving Self-Test contained in Chapter 3, you have measured your present state of well-being. I'd recommend repeating this test every two to three months to gauge your physical, mental, and spiritual health progress and in your training as *a healer of yourself.*

In the process of healing your body along with your asthmatic lungs, the ultimate objective is the following state of physical and environmental well-being:

PHYSICAL HEALTH
High energy and vitality
- Freedom from, or high adaptability to, pain, dysfunction, and disability
- A strong immune system
- A body that feels light, balanced, strong, flexible, and has good aerobic capacity
- Ability to meet physical challenges and perform exceptionally
- Full capacity of all five senses and a healthy libido

ENVIRONMENTAL HEALTH

Harmony with your environment (neither harming nor being harmed)
- Awareness of your connectedness with nature
- Feeling grounded—comfort and security within your surroundings
- Respect and appreciation for your home, the Earth, and all of her inhabitants
- Contact with the Earth; breathing healthy air; drinking pure water; eating uncontaminated food; exposure to the sun, fire, or candlelight; immersion in warm water (all on a daily basis)

HOLISTIC MEDICAL TREATMENT AND PREVENTION

To begin to restore your body to a heightened state of harmony and to correct the present imbalance manifested by your asthmatic lungs, your *primary goals* are:

1. **To heal the mucous membrane lining your lungs, nose, and sinuses**
2. **To strengthen and restore balance to your immune system**
3. **To address each of the possible causes of your asthma**

In meeting these goals you can potentially cure your asthma while you're healing your life. The word *cure* refers to a physical problem, while *heal* has to do with the condition of your life. However, it is possible to cure your dysfunctional lungs but still be living an imbalanced life; or, conversely, you may feel whole, balanced, at peace with your life while still experiencing some degree of asthma. In essence, *this holistic approach will provide you with the potential to do both—cure asthma and heal your life—while you are engaged in the process of loving and nurturing your inflamed, hypersensitive, and hyperreactive mucous membrane along with the rest of you.* As you begin, you should now keep in mind the image of a pink, vibrant, glistening (covered with a thin, clear mucus) mucous membrane lining your lungs, nose, and sinuses. (If mental imagery is difficult for you, then look in the mirror and pull your lower lip down. The inner lining of your lip closely resembles a healthy respiratory mucous membrane.) This healing vision can be expanded in any way you'd like. But it is important to keep it in mind as often as you can, since it will help you to stay focused on the goal of your treatment and, even more important, to make that *vision become a reality.*

Think of the Asthma Survival Program as *a personalized course in self-healing and optimal well-being.* In this and the following chapters, you will be provided with a "curriculum" or, if you prefer, a "prescription" for improving six components of health while treating each of the primary causes of asthma. I have tried to simplify each component and have suggested "exercises" to help you find your own path to a greater level of physical, environmental, mental, emotional, spiritual, and social fitness. These exercises must be practiced regularly in order to be effective. (However, if after giving it a fair trial, a particular exercise feels too uncomfortable to you, then stop.) If you are willing to be patient—remember, it took years for you to develop your current state of health—I promise that you will feel better, although I cannot guarantee you will cure your asthma. Yet your chances for doing so are far greater using this approach than if you strictly adhered to the conventional medical treatment, with its chief objective being the *management* of the condition while preventing and treating the symptoms. Holistic medicine is not an alternative but a complement to what you are already doing for your asthma. It is also the most therapeutically sound and cost-effective approach to the treatment of chronic disease that I've found in nearly thirty years of practicing medicine. By taking responsibility for your own health, you become not only your own healer but a highly skilled practitioner of preventive medicine. You'll learn what *causes* your wheezing, coughing, and shortness of breath, and will be able to make well-informed choices regarding your asthmatic condition. You're also a pioneer of sorts, since the holistic self-care model presented on the following pages will soon become an essential part of the foundation of primary-care medicine. Keep in mind that although this is a course with a lot of homework, there are no exams or grades, no mistakes or failures, just a series of valuable lessons to help you feel more fully alive. Enjoy yourself! What do you have to lose?

The foundation of the physical aspect of holistic medical treatment is to love and nurture your body with safe, gentle, and effective therapies. You should have a much better idea of how to do that, especially for your respiratory tract, after reading this chapter. Remember that the essentials of the physical and environmental health components of the Asthma Survival Program can also be found in Chapter 1.

Symptom Treatment

I recommend beginning the Asthma Survival Program with an aggressive approach to treating the symptoms of your asthma. This includes consulting with your physician and making sure that you have treated your condition with the best methods that conventional medicine has to offer, even if they provide only temporary and symptomatic relief. It is also essential that you determine if the benefits of that treatment outweigh the liabilities. For instance, bronchodilators and anti–inflammatories (corticosteroids) may cause dependence and depress the immune system. If you've decided that the risks of continuing this course of symptom treatment are too great or that it's not giving you effective relief, there are several options that will be offered to you in this chapter.

As you begin the Asthma Survival Program, it is helpful to rate each of your symptoms on a scale of 1 to 10, with 1 being an almost incapacitating symptom and 10 being perfectly normal (no symptom). You can use the Symptom Chart (page 62) and rate yourself at the end of each week. It provides you with both an objective (most of the symptoms can be measured objectively—you can either see, hear, or feel them) and a subjective (energy level, emotions) means of monitoring your progress. You don't need anyone else or a pulmonary function test to tell

Symptom Chart

Began Asthma Survival Program on _____
Rate Symptoms from 1 (worst) to 10 (best = normal)

SYMPTOM	BEGIN ___ (date)	END WEEK 1	END WEEK 2	END WEEK 3	END WEEK 4	END WEEK 5	END WEEK 6	END WEEK 7	END WEEK 8	END WEEK 9	END WEEK 10	END WEEK 11	END WEEK 12
Shortness of breath													
Wheezing													
Cough—dry													
Cough—wet/mucusy													
Head congestion (fullness)													
Nasal congestion (stuffy nose)													
Postnasal drip													
Headache													
Yellow/green mucus (from nose)													
Yellow/green mucus (back of throat)													
Sneezing													
Itching: nose, throat													

SYMPTOM	BEGIN ___ (date)	END WEEK 1	END WEEK 2	END WEEK 3	END WEEK 4	END WEEK 5	END WEEK 6	END WEEK 7	END WEEK 8	END WEEK 9	END WEEK 10	END WEEK 11	END WEEK 12
Ear congestion (ears plugged up)													
Sore throat													
Swollen glands (in neck)													
Fatigue (rate energy level)													
Avg no. of hrs. sleep													
Other symptoms:													
Medications: (pharmaceutical drugs) (use a "√" if still taking drug)													
Vitamins/herbs supplements (use a "√" if still taking)													

you how well you're doing. Please add any symptoms to this chart that are not listed but that often cause you discomfort. Because so many asthmatics also suffer from sinusitis and allergies, and the Asthma and Sinus Survival Programs overlap to a great extent, the preceding chart lists the most common symptoms of all three conditions—that is, a Respiratory Disease Symptom Chart.

Physical and Environmental Health Recommendations for Asthma

1. AIR AND BREATHING

There is nothing more important to human health and survival than the quality of the air we breathe. Since air pollution, both indoor and outdoor, is a primary cause for the chronic irritation and inflammation of the mucous membranes lining the entire respiratory tract, then breathing healthy air is an essential component of the Asthma Survival Program. It is the job of the nose and sinuses to protect the lungs. They do so by functioning as the body's:

1. Air filter—they remove particles, pollen, smoke, mold, animal dander, bacteria, and viruses
2. Humidifier—they moisten dry air
3. Temperature regulator—they warm cold air and cool extremely hot air

If the nose and sinuses are not functioning at peak efficiency, or if they're congested or infected with allergies, a cold, or a sinus infection, then the lungs are at greater risk for developing asthma or bronchitis. Since the health of the lungs is so closely connected to that of the nose and sinuses, the following recommendations for creating a healthy indoor environment will benefit all three parts of the respiratory tract.

Optimal Air Quality

The first step in improving both your physical and environmental health is to change the quality of the indoor air you're breathing—in essence, to create healing rather than harmful or irritating air. All of the recommendations mentioned in this section are helpful. But at the very least I would start with a negative-ion generator in your bedroom and, if you can afford it, in your workplace as well. Within three to four weeks I would add a warm-mist humidifier in the bedroom (especially during the winter months), along with plants in the house, an effective furnace filter, followed by air duct and carpet cleaning. If the expense does not deter you, then a central humidifier installed on the furnace will complete your indoor air enhancement program. You may not create optimal indoor air, but you'll be close.

Air quality is rated by clarity (freedom from pollutants), humidity (ideal is between 35 and 55 percent), temperature (between 65° and 85°F), oxygen content (21 percent of total volume and 100 percent saturation), and negative ion content (3,000 to 6,000 .001-micron ions per cubic centimeter). Air that is clean, moist, warm, oxygen-rich, and high in negative ions is the healthiest air a human being can breathe.

Not only are we dependent on oxygen for survival, but every part of the human body thrives with a maximum supply of oxygen. If your respiratory tract is defective because of a nasal, sinus, or lung ailment, or if the amount of oxygen available in the air is relatively low—air that is high in carbon monoxide and/or other pollutants, air at higher altitudes (oxygen content decreases by over 3 percent every thousand feet above sea level), or stale indoor air—your body is receiving less than its optimal requirement of oxygen. Scientists report that the oxygen content of the air in some polluted cities is as low as 8 percent instead of the normal 21 percent. If you live in a polluted high-altitude city such as Denver, Salt Lake City, or Albuquerque, then your body is receiving far less oxygen than it needs for optimal function.

Negative ions are air molecules that have excess electrons. Negative ions vitalize or freshen the air we breathe by removing unhealthy particles. The earth itself is a natural negative-ion generator. Health spas have always been located in areas high in negative ions (3,000 to 20,000 per cubic centimeter of air), such as along seacoasts, near rushing streams and waterfalls, in mountainous areas, and in pine forests (pine needles cause negative ions to be generated in the surrounding air). Although unproven, there is speculation that negative ions increase the sweeping motion of the cilia on the respiratory mucosa, and subsequently enhance the movement of mucus and the clearing or filtering of inhaled pollutants. Unfortunately, there is very little research on the effect of negative ions on the respiratory tract. Two studies were performed in the 1960s in Israel that indicated negative ions had a beneficial effect on asthmatics, but to my knowledge there has been no recent research. However, what has been conclusively proven is that negative ions are effective air cleaners. They attract dust, smoke, mold, pollen, bacteria, and viruses, all of which have a positive charge. The heavier combined particle (the negative ion plus the pollen, etc.) then falls from the air to the ground and is removed from the breathing space. Negative ions also have been shown to help reduce pain, heal burns, suppress mold and bacterial growth, and stimulate plant growth, and they contribute greatly to our sense of well-being and comfort. Positive ions, on the other hand, are air molecules lacking electrons. Pollen can carry fifty or more positive charges per grain of pollen. This positive charge slows the cilia and the clearing of mucus, and in so doing can cause some degree of nasal congestion. Most man-made pollutants result from combustion processes (auto/truck exhaust, smokestacks, cigarette smoke, etc.), which leave the pollutants with a positive charge. Heating and ventilation systems tend to produce air containing an excess of positive ions. Aircraft cabins have been tested and found to contain an excessively high amount of positive ions. This obviously contributes to the "stuffy" feeling of airplane air, and also helps to explain why so many of my patients have developed colds and sinus infections following air travel.

The negative ion content of indoor air can be as low as 10 to 200 negative ions per cubic centimeter. This is considered to be "ion-depleted" air and is a significant component of "sick-building syndrome." Ion-depleted air is also created by heating/cooling systems; window air conditioners; air cleaners (including HEPA filters), which "scrub" negative ions from the air; and the screens of television sets and computers, which have a high positive charge that draws negative ions out of the air and neutralizes them. Most of the factors in our environment responsible for depleting the beneficial negative ions also produce an excess of unhealthy positive ions.

The majority of Americans spend 90 percent of their time indoors, where, the EPA says, the air can be as much as 100 times more polluted than outdoor air. Few of us live in clean, moist environments that are warm year-round; even fewer live in the mountains, on a beach, or in the woods. For the 92 million people whose lungs, sinuses, and noses are already adversely affected from breathing unhealthy air, and for anyone else who wants to enjoy optimum health, here are some ways to minimize the risks of breathing poor-quality air and to prevent and treat asthma, sinusitis, and allergies.

Healthy Homes

Where we live, work, play, or otherwise spend our time is critical to our health. If you are considering a move, you should look for a home in a location that minimizes the impact of outdoor air pollution or in a city or town that has minimal air pollution. If you have the freedom to choose, avoid the following regions: southern California, the Northeast, and the Texas Gulf Coast. The healthiest air can be found along the West Coast (with the distinct exception of the Los Angeles metropolitan area and southward), rural areas along the Gulf Coast (other than Texas), and the west coast of Florida.

If you are contemplating the construction of a new home, the concept of *ecological architecture* could help considerably in creating a healthy environment. *Ecology* is defined in Webster's *New World Dictionary* as "the branch of biology that deals with the relationship between living organisms and their environment." Used as a modifier for the word *architecture,* it simply means the design of a dwelling that is sensitive to human health and gentle to the earth. Once we have considered the microclimate and the site, our biological needs, behavior patterns, and, most important, our budgetary limitations, nature will then dictate the design. Self-sufficiency through use of sun, air, earth, and water for heating, cooling, ventilation, and even electrical power is a realistic goal of an ecological design.

Common objectives regarding construction methods and materials include:

- Avoiding the use of plastic or other materials made of toxic ingredients that harmfully outgas (give off toxins and/or fumes) in the indoor environment
- Using nontoxic natural materials in preference to synthetic materials
- Designing with concern for sensitivities, allergies, or chronic health problems
- Being aware that nature's ecologic sustainability and well-being should not be diminished by what is built
- Taking the responsibility to conceive, design, build, and furnish a home or building to a "healthy home" ecological ethic.

This is a holistic approach emphasizing the ecological bond between site and architecture. Preservation and wise use of our planet's resources in construction and throughout the lifetime of a home is fundamental to ecological design. For the asthmatic allergy or sinus sufferer, a home must be clean, moist, warm, and oxygen- and negative ion–rich. The fact that it is designed in harmony with the atmosphere and the earth makes this an environmentally healthy concept.

I fully appreciate that most readers of this book will neither move nor design their own home as a result of what they read here. However, I want to present as many environmental treatment options as possible. Each can potentially benefit your asthma, producing a profound impact on your overall state of health and ultimately your quality of life. Fortunately, technology has made it possible to create an oasis of healthy indoor air in your own home, so you won't have to move or build a new home. In the desert an oasis provides water. In the sea of hazardous air in which we live, a *healthy home* or business can provide an oasis in which to breathe life-enhancing air.

Solving the problem of indoor air pollution entails both treatment and prevention. There is a company in Denver, Healthy Habitats, that has been on the leading edge of this field for over twelve years. The owner of the company, Carl Grimes, has worked with me and a number of my patients to transform our unhealthy homes and offices into healthy ones. The procedures and techniques he employs adhere to the following guidelines:

- Prevention—avoid bringing pollutants into the home and workplace.
- Identify the source and develop a plan for isolating or removing the pollutant from the "breathing zone" or the surrounding area from which you obtain your breathing air—for example, an infant's breathing zone includes the floor and carpeting.
- Reduce ambient pollution with ventilation, filtration, and ionization.

Grimes considers the three primary sources of pollution to be:

- Particulates—dust, pollen, dander, construction debris, and smoke
- Microorganisms—bacteria, viruses, molds, and dust mites
- Chemicals and gases—personal care products, cleaning products, office equipment, and building/construction materials. (Refer to Table 2.1, pages 33–34.)

The type of treatment depends on the type of pollution. For example, HEPA filtration might be used for particulates, charcoal might be used for chemicals and gases, and the drying of a wet crawl space could be the best option for eliminating microbes. Ozone has also been effective for persistent microorganisms; however, when a home is cleaned with ozone, the residents are advised to vacate the premises for two to three days. Chemical and gaseous pollution is harder to avoid than particulate matter and may be a significant reason for the increase in asthma. Although activated charcoal filters may be effective for removing toxic gases (formaldehyde is the most common gas found in homes), a simpler strategy involves the use of houseplants known to absorb gases from the air (refer to page 78).

Molds are rapidly becoming one of America's chief health hazards and one of the leading causes of the dramatic increase in asthma, allergies, and chronic sinusitis during the past twenty years. In addition to the overuse of antibiotics, many of us are being exposed daily to high levels of mold. The problem has resulted primarily from modern home design—more airtight, with air-conditioning and heating systems recirculating contaminated air; materials used; and, most important, *water leaks.* Molds can grow wherever it's damp, so it's important to quickly fix any leaks, regularly clean air ducts and furnace filters, be on the lookout for discoloration of walls or ceilings and any unusual odors, and empty (daily) and clean (weekly) humidifiers on a regular basis.

Several excellent books are available on the subject of healthy homes. I recommend the following: *Starting Points for a Healthy Habitat,* by Carl Grimes (Healthy Habitats); *The Nontoxic Home and Office* by Debra Lynn Dadd (Jeremy P. Tarcher, Inc.); *The Healthy House* by John Bower (Lyle Stuart, Inc.); and *Your Home, Your Health and Well-Being* by David Rousseau (Ten Speed Press).

Air Cleaners and Negative-Ion Generators

As many as one million hospital admissions a year are attributed to poor indoor air quality. In recent years, as the EPA and private health organizations have publicized the problem of indoor air pollution, we have seen a proliferation of types of air cleaners; today there are almost as many as there are indoor air pollutants. According to Michael Berry, Ph.D., former manager of the EPA's Indoor Air Project, the most potentially harmful pollutants are radon and the "biologicals," including pollen, mold, plant spores, dust mites, bacteria, and viruses. The pollutants most harmful to the respiratory tract are less than one micron in size. Regardless of their origin, size, or health-damaging effects, air pollutants can be described as free-floating particles in the air. Figure 4.1 shows the specific size ranges of the most common pollutants. The unit of measurement used for tiny air particles is the micron. An average hair strand is 100 microns thick, and about 400 one-micron particles would fit into the dot over the *i* in the word *micron*. The primary job of air cleaners is to re-

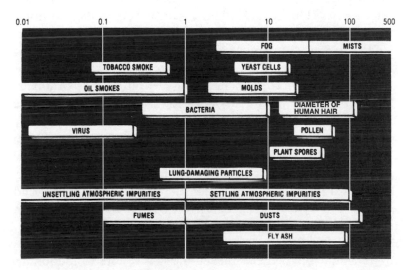

FIGURE 4.1   *Relative size of common air contaminants.*

move as many of these particles as possible, the biologicals as well as the combustion products, particulates, chemicals, fumes, and odors. (See Table 2.1, pages 33–34.) Radon, if present, requires the sealing of basement cracks and improvement of basement ventilation. Most air cleaners do not remove radon from the air. However, some air cleaners with high particle-removal efficiency (HEPA, etc.) can remove some of the radon "daughters" (attached radon) that are in particulate form. A study at the Harvard School of Public Health determined that a negative-ion generator is a highly effective means of removing the attached fraction of radon (the radon daughters), although it does not reduce the unattached (gaseous) fraction of radon.

The strategy for solving the problem of indoor air pollution involves air cleaning and improved ventilation. Air-cleaning devices can include furnace filters, portable standalone units, and negative-ion generators. The efficiency of air cleaners is evaluated by their ability to filter a certain percentage of a certain size of pollutant. The HEPA filter (an acronym for high-efficiency particulate arrestor) removes 97 percent of all 0.3-micron particulates and larger. This includes pollen, plant spores, most animal dander, dust, wood, tobacco smoke, fumes, bacteria, and some viruses. This type of filter is standard equipment for most hospital operating suites, and is found in many of the more expensive freestanding air cleaners. It requires a strong fan or a booster fan to move air through it due to its increased efficiency.

The ULPA (ultra-low penetrating air) filters were originally created to purify the air in semiconductor clean rooms. The Bionaire company has now made this new technology available to clean the air in homes. ULPA air purifiers are equipped with a superfine filter that removes a remarkable 99.999 percent of all airborne particles as small as 0.1 micron. The filter traps such allergens as tobacco smoke, pollen, dust, dust mites, mold, and bacteria. For best performance, it is recommended that ULPA filters be changed every six months to one year.

Negative-ion generators were originally designed to restore a more natural and beneficial level of negative ions to indoor air. In the course of their use for biological benefit, it was discovered that free-floating ions quickly attach to airborne particles and cause them to agglomerate and precipitate from the air, or be drawn to grounded surfaces such as walls and metal surfaces. Ionizers are highly effective air cleaners, removing particles as small as .001 micron, which would include viruses, molds, dust, pollen, cigarette smoke, and all other airborne particulate pollutants. Compared to air cleaners with fans or blowers, ionizers are more likely to be operated full-time since they are totally silent (no fan) and consume only pennies' worth of electricity per month.

However, in order to increase the speed with which an ionizer cleans the air, many manufacturers produce ionizers with excessive ion output. This has two undesirable effects: (1) The ion density established by these ionizers exceeds by many times the natural range found outdoors, resulting in much the same adverse effects as breathing air with too few negative ions. A well-designed negative-ion generator will generate enough ions to be effective but will not exceed an upper limit that would make it biologically undesirable. (2) An excessively high ion density also causes a significant amount of pollutants to be driven to the walls and other grounded surfaces, resulting in the buildup of a dirty residue. Again, a well-designed ion generator will minimize such "plating," and this effect can be further reduced by placing the ionizer at least two feet from the nearest wall.

It has been my good fortune, and that of my patients, to have worked with a "pioneer" in negative-ion technology. For nearly thirty years Rex Coppom, owner of Electrofilter Technologies in Longmont, Colorado, has been developing state-of-the-art negative-ion generators. For almost eight years many of my patients have been using his Sinus Survival Air Vitalizer, a small unit that cleans the air of a 150- to 200-square-foot room and whose self-regulation feature enables it to maintain an ideal level of negative ions (3,000 to 6,000 per cubic centimeter). It costs $150, considerably less than the average price of a HEPA room air cleaner, which is somewhat less efficient in its cleaning capacity and has no negative ions. I have received many testimonials about its beneficial effects—fewer allergy and asthma attacks, dramatic headache relief, diminished nasal congestion, cessation of snoring, better sleep, more energy, general feelings of well-being, and diminished odor and symptoms resulting from secondhand cigarette smoke. I was amazed at how quickly it cleared the smoke from my kitchen during an oven-cleaning session that went somewhat awry. Ionization equipment is currently available for automobiles and aircraft cabins—both of which have far less than optimum air.

Electronic air cleaners (both central and freestanding) produce positive ions as they filter the air. On their first day of operation they are 85 percent efficient on all 1-micron and larger particles, but in order to maintain that efficiency they require cleaning every two weeks. For most of us, this makes them impractical and inconvenient. They also produce ozone, which can be a potential health hazard.

To obtain a furnace filter, go to a hardware or building-supply store. Many of them carry the 3M pleated filter, under the brand name Filtret. These are excellent furnace filters and cost about $15. They should be replaced every one to two months during the winter and while central air conditioners are being run regularly. They are far more efficient than the $2 to $4 varieties found in supermarkets. There are several other brands of pleated furnace filters that are similar in efficiency to 3M.

The Du Pont Wizard dustcloth is an interesting product that does a better job of dusting than can be obtained from liquid or spray dust cleaners. They are used dry, can be washed, and cost $2.

Air Duct Cleaning

When the air duct system of my thirteen-year-old home was cleaned for the first time, I was amazed at what emanated from the ducts after two hours of high-intensity vacuuming. I thought to myself, "It's no wonder I suffered with sinus problems for so long!" If the air ducts are filthy, it is nearly impossible for your furnace filter to clean the air in your home. After the air is filtered, it still has to travel through the ducts before you breathe it. I recommend air duct cleaning as part of the environmental treatment program. Depending on the size of your home, an air duct cleaning service, using good equipment, could cost between $200 and $250. To find this type of company in your city, look in the Yellow Pages under "Furnaces, Cleaning and Repairing."

Carpet Cleaning

Carpets are one of the most common sources of indoor air pollutants. They are excellent traps and hold on to dust, pollen, and microorganisms. While this helps to keep those particles out of the breathing zone, their gradual accumulation can become great enough to create a sustainable culture of bacteria, yeast, dust mites, and mold. In fact, many allergists recommend that their patients dispose of all their carpets.

While it is true that carpets harbor pollutants, it is possible to keep them clean. This poses a challenge to the homemaker. Conventional vacuum cleaners are designed to remove and retain the visible dirt, which means particles greater than 10 microns. Most of the particles and microorganisms that are too small to be seen are also smaller than the pores in the vacuum cleaner bag. This allows most of them to blow through the bag and into the room, settling back onto the carpets and furniture. If a forced-air heating system is running, the airborne particles can be drawn into the air ducts, contributing to their contamination as well. Also, as the bag fills, airflow decreases, causing uneven cleaning.

To prevent these problems, I suggest a vacuum cleaner that uses either a HEPA-type filter or water capture. Either one removes even subvisible dust and bacteria from the air. The water-capture types also have a continuously maximum airflow because they won't clog like a bag or filter. Both of these vacuums are expensive, costing between $500 and $1,000.

However, there is a much less expensive alternative. Dupont Hysurf vacuum cleaner bags have 1-micron pores and cost only $5. They appear to have the equivalent cleaning efficiency of the $500-plus "allergy" vacuum cleaners. Their major drawback is that they are difficult to find. Some janitorial supply houses and medical supply stores have them. They can also be obtained from Sinus Survival Products.

Many people have their carpets professionally cleaned. However, due to their chemical composition, the most common cleaning agents are often worse than having dirty carpets. Alcohols, petroleum distillates, ammonia, dry-cleaning substances, and scents often cause headaches, mental "fuzziness," lethargy, and a general feeling of discomfort. Cleaning-agent residues may often cause respiratory irritation.

Before contracting with a carpet cleaner, check his references and insist on a nonscented cleaning agent that uses no petroleum distillates, alcohol, ammonia, or dry-cleaning-type chemicals or enzymes, and has no suds that can be left in the carpet. Check his work to be sure he leaves no damp areas. This ensures maximum removal of all agents and enhances drying time. If the carpet stays wet for several days, bacteria and molds can grow rapidly.

Ventilation and Plants

All indoor spaces, whether residential, commercial, industrial, or recreational, require some type of ventilation to provide breathable air for occupants, to furnish combustion air for cooking and heating, and to remove stale air filled with toxins and particulates. Commercial buildings are required by code to have even more efficient ventilation systems than residences. The American Society of Heating, Refrigerating and Air-Conditioning Engineers (ASHRAE) says that air should be replaced at the rate of 15 cubic feet per minute per person, but most systems fall below this minimum standard.

Improving ventilation will help relieve indoor air pollution as long as the outdoor air isn't dirtier than the air it is replacing. Local pollution sources, such as fumes from toxic waste leakage, wood burning, a neighboring industrial plant, a heavily trafficked highway, or crop spraying can render outdoor air unacceptable for indoor ventilation. Several days a year Los Angeles residents are advised to keep all windows and doors closed and ventilation ducts shut to prevent the heavily polluted outdoor air from entering homes and businesses. In areas like this it becomes a challenge to balance the health benefit of highly oxygenated outdoor air and the liability of the pollutants that come with it. Outdoor aerobic exercise presents a similar dilemma. If you live in a heavily polluted environment, I recommend exercising outside and ventilating your home and office well when outdoor air is good, but exercise indoors and keep windows and doors closed during periods of heavy pollution.

Air-conditioning systems are a helpful means of ventilation for people with asthma and allergy problems. These systems remove excess moisture from the air, lowering its temperature. In less humid conditions there is a reduction of molds and spores, and with the windows closed there is also a marked decrease in pollen from the outdoors. Air-conditioning, however, does deplete negative ions from the air.

Natural cross-ventilation is effective in reducing indoor air pollution if the placement of the intake vents is low and the outlets for the flow-through air are high. Operable windows on commercial buildings and a good location for the outdoor air intake—away from garage entrances or loading docks—are also important factors in improving indoor air quality. Mechanical ventilation with exhaust fans can certainly help in removing indoor pollutants, but such fans are most efficient when used in a confined space. Private offices or single-occupant rooms where smoking, cooking, and other fume-producing activities take place are ideal environments for mechanical ventilation.

Rooms producing commercial toxic or odoriferous fumes; spaces subject to bacterial and viral contamination, such as rest rooms; and indoor areas that present specific respiratory hazards all need optimized ventilation. Mold is a special problem in moist conditions. Adequate ventilation along with sunshine can help to reduce moisture and subsequently suppress mold.

The technology of ventilation can be complex, but the basic principle of displacing interior air with outdoor air and increasing the rate of fresh airflow is critical to treating the problem of indoor air pollution. Besides natural cross-ventilation and exhaust fans, other devices used to enhance ventilation and indoor air quality are air-to-air heat exchangers, makeup air units, attic fans, vortex fans, and ceiling fans. Remember that even if the "fresh" air is filthy, an effective air cleaner combined with good ventilation is still a winning combination.

Adequate ventilation not only helps reduce indoor air pollution but is the primary source of indoor oxygen. Plants can offer an aesthetically pleasant secondary source in addition to their ability to remove toxic gases from the air. Although the oxygen output from indoor plants is not great, plants with large leaf surfaces that grow rapidly are capable of enhancing air quality. Attached greenhouses and atria filled with plants that effectively absorb carbon dioxide and oxygenate the air (spider plants do this very well) can improve the indoor environment while humidifying the air.

In the early 1990s, studies conducted at the John Stennis Space Center in Mississippi showed that plants can also act as effective filters. Former NASA scientist Bill C. Wolverton, Ph.D., has spent the past thirty years studying the ability of plants to clear volatile organic chemicals from indoor air. Wolverton predicts that within twenty years plants will be governmentally mandated in new buildings as a matter of public health.

According to the EPA, the most plentiful of the organic chemicals in the average indoor environment is formaldehyde. It is released from a host of household furnishings, including synthetic carpeting, particleboard (used to make bookcases, desks, and tables), foam insulation, upholstery, curtains, and even so-called air fresheners. Common houseplants such as chrysanthemums, striped dracaena, dwarf date palms, and especially Boston ferns are excellent filters for removing formaldehyde. Spider plants are also effective in removing carbon monoxide; areca palms are best at filtering xylene, the second-most-prevalent indoor organic chemical; and English ivy is good for filtering benzene, ranked third on the EPA's list. Aloe vera, philodendron, pothos, and ficus were also found to reduce levels of organic chemicals.

The Foliage for Clean Air Council, a communications clear-inghouse for information on the use of foliage to improve indoor air quality, recommends a minimum of two plants per 100 square feet of floor space in an average home with eight- to ten-foot ceilings.

Plants can help improve indoor air as oxygenators, filters, and humidifiers.

Prevention

Prevention of indoor air pollution involves eliminating pollutants at the source. Doctors who specialize in environmental medicine and some allergists can do skin and blood tests to help you identify pollutants to which you are particularly sensitive or allergic. These doctors are not always easy to find, nor are the tests always definitive, but they can help. With the use of environmentally sensitive architectural principles, a healthier home can be created. A major preventive strategy is the use of interior materials that emit no pollutants. Natural products such as wood, cotton, and metals are preferable to the lower-cost synthetic materials such as particleboard, fiberboard, polyester, and plastics.

Choosing to forgo a fireplace or wood-burning stove would be helpful, as would using a high-efficiency furnace with a sealed combustion unit to vent exhaust gases to the outside. Switch to nontoxic cleaning substances, including ordinary soap, vinegar, zephiran, and Air Therapy. (You can find a listing of such cleaners in *Nontoxic, Natural, & Earthwise,* by Debra Lynn Dadd.) Smoking should be relegated to the outdoors or to a well-ventilated enclosed space. If radon levels exceed the acceptable EPA standard of 4 picoCuries per liter of air, radon-control measures should be implemented. Formaldehyde from insulation can be eliminated by using the substitutes of cellulose and white fiberglass insulation.

Humidification

According to Dr. Marshall Plaut, chief of the asthma and allergy branch at the National Institute of Allergy and Infectious Diseases (part of NIH), "Dry air triggers asthma and nasal congestion." I, too, have been convinced for quite some time that dry air, and especially cold and dry air, is a major contributor to asthma, sinusitis, bronchitis. As a chronic irritant to the sensitive nasal mucous membrane, dry air can also contribute to a greater susceptibility to allergies. Studies on patients with allergic rhinitis have shown that warm, moist air can reduce nasal congestion and other allergy symptoms.

Optimum indoor air quality requires air containing between 35 and 55 percent relative humidity. Moisture provided by room humidifiers can greatly benefit anyone with a respiratory condition. These humidifiers are most helpful in the winter, even in humid, cold-weather climates, because most heating systems dry the indoor air considerably. However, if you are sensitive to mold and believe that exposure to mold is a primary trigger of your asthma, then I would be more cautious about using a humidifier.

Room humidifiers, also called tabletop models, have sufficient capacity to humidify a medium- to large-size room. Each type has some drawbacks. Ultrasonic models can emit an irritating white dust. So can cool mist models, which require the use of distilled water or an expensive demineralization cartridge, unless you have very soft water. Steam-mist models, also called vaporizers, can scald if you get too close to the mist they produce or if you tip them over by accident. Evaporative models, the most prevalent type, can become a breeding ground for bacteria. The warm-mist units are my first choice. They produce a mist just slightly warmer than room air, use tap water, require no filter, and are able to kill bacteria. Their only drawback may be that they use more electricity than the other types. Most humidifiers are quiet and very effective in producing a moist environment in an enclosed space. They are available in pharmacies, department stores, and hardware stores under a variety of brand names. The one I know best and with which I have enjoyed excellent results is the Bionaire–Clear Mist 5 (CMP-5). It quietly yet powerfully puts out warm moisture, can cover an area of up to 1,600 square feet, and is relatively easy to clean. The Kenmore Warm Mist is the identical unit, and it is available at most Sears stores. These units cost about $125. Although the ideal humidifier has probably not yet been designed, I've recently tried the Slant/Fin GF-200. This warm–mist humidifier uses ultraviolet germicidal technology to produce 99.999 percent germ-free mist. It costs under $100. The tabletop humidifiers can cost from $30 to $125.

The larger humidifiers, called consoles, can humidify an average-size house, cost from $100 to $200, and are all the evaporative type. Although I've had no personal experience with these, I know that *Consumer Reports* has given a high rating to the Bionaire W-6S, as well as to the Toastmaster 3435 and Emerson HD850.

Central or in-duct humidifiers, those that attach to the furnace, are more convenient but often do not humidify an individual room as well as a portable humidifier can when the door to the room is closed. In the past the major problem with central humidifiers has been that most of them were the reservoir type, with a tray of standing water that breeds mold and bacteria. I recommend the flow-through type of central humidifier— for example, Aprilaire or General—which eliminates the stagnant water problem and is easy to maintain. Depending on the model, size of your home, and installation, this humidifier would probably cost about $250 to $650.

Humidifiers are not the only option for moisturizing your home. The installation of waterfalls, indoor spas, and swimming pools will all add a lot of moisture to the house, but of course they are expensive to install and maintain. It may surprise you to learn that even the moisture from human breath and sweat, along with that from cooking, baths, showers, and plants, adds significantly to a home's humidity. If your bedroom is dry, hang a wet towel on a hanger in the room.

If you rarely suffer jolts of static electricity when you touch metal objects such as doorknobs, then the air in your home is probably humid enough. For a more precise test, you'll need a hygrometer. You can find these humidity measuring devices at most hardware stores. The one I've been using is the Bionaire Climate Check, a digital device that measures both temperature and humidity.

Breathing

Oxygen is the most critical nutrient for every cell in the body. It is literally the "spark of life" needed to provide energy for every basic bodily function. Breathing is our constant and immediate connection to life: We can go days without water, weeks without food, but only minutes without oxygen. We begin life with our first breath, and end it with our last. During our adult life we normally breathe about 23,000 times a day without ever giving much thought to this miraculous process. Because respiration, synchronized with heartbeat, is an automatic function, we are seldom aware of how we breathe, or attempt to breathe more efficiently or healthfully, until we are confronted with the crisis of having great difficulty breathing. The frightening, at times terrifying, onset of an asthmatic attack instantaneously alerts us to the vital need for oxygen. Suddenly you become intimately aware of your own breath, your heart rate, muscle tension, your anxiety and fear. Your breath is labored and you feel yourself fighting to breathe to save your life! The harder you struggle to breathe, the more rapid and shallow your breaths become, decreasing the available amount of both oxygen and carbon dioxide. (As you'll soon learn, carbon dioxide is more than simply a waste product of respiration.) This situation then increases the need for oxygen in your tissues, which triggers spasm in the bronchioles, which in turn causes wheezing. It can become a vicious cycle leading to long-term dysfunction and drug dependency. (If you're uncertain if you've ever experienced asthma, then try breathing through a drinking straw, which can simulate the degree of breathing difficulty accompanying an asthma attack.) Breathing techniques, along with judicious use of medication and natural therapies, can help to break the cycle of labored breathing relatively quickly and restore normal function. This can then provide the opportunity to reduce medication to a minimum.

According to recent research, overbreathing might be a primary factor in triggering an asthmatic attack. Hyperventilation can decrease carbon dioxide, which ultimately affects utilization of oxygen in the cells. Medical professor Konstantin Buteyko, a Russian researcher, has performed extensive experiments in Russia for over forty-five years finding that virtually all asthma patients overbreathe on a regular basis. This led him to the controversial theory that hyperventilation is a primary *cause* of asthma! He defines hyperventilation as the habitual inhalation of more than 4 to 6 liters of air per minute—considered to be the normal rate of respiration. It is the equivalent of 8 to 12 breaths per minute, with each breath being the equivalent of a pint of air, or about two gallons per minute. In contrast, a person practiced in slow, rhythmic breathing may inhale 5 liters over a 3-minute period, or a rate between 3 and 4 breaths per minute. With asthma, it can be as high as 10 to 15 liters during a 1-minute period, as much as 20 to 30 breaths per minute. This type of breathing lowers carbon dioxide excessively.

Professor Buteyko recognized carbon dioxide as not just a waste product, but an important chemical regulator that is essential for the *utilization* of oxygen in the cells. Chronic overbreathing creates a deficiency of carbon dioxide, which increases bronchospasm and decreases *available* oxygen. By teaching patients techniques of slow, periodic underbreathing he found that he could effect a significant reduction in asthma symptoms in 90 percent of his patients. Teresa Hale, founder of the highly regarded Hale Clinic in London (the United Kingdom's largest holistic medical clinic with over one hundred practitioners, including thirty M.D.s), has confirmed Buteyko's findings and claims his breathing techniques have produced dramatic reductions in asthma symptoms in just five days. She, too, found that it worked for 90 percent of their patients. To date, over one million people in the former Soviet Union have applied this technique with similar results. In October 2000, the *Journal of Asthma* reported that Australian researchers, Dr. M. J. Abramson and colleagues of the Alfred Hospital in Prahan, Victoria, did a placebo-controlled study on thirty-six patients who were given an instructional video on the Buteyko Method, watched it daily for four weeks, and practiced the breathing techniques. The treatment group showed significant improvement in quality of life and reduction of bronchodilator use. (For more in-depth information about Buteyko's Method, refer to the book *Breathing Free* by Teresa Hale.)

Twenty years ago, Dr. Todd Nelson learned breathing techniques for asthma from one of naturopathic medicine's pioneers, Dr. Bernard Jensen. His techniques emphasized breathing out over breathing in—similar to Buteyko's method. Although at the time it seemed somewhat confusing to him, he noticed that his patients who practiced these breathing techniques consistently improved! Today, a growing number of researchers and practitioners are concluding that breathing techniques that emphasize the out breath, while breathing slowly and through the nose, are highly effective. While doing the research for this book, we found that two other physicians, Richard Firshein, D.O., and Ron Roberts, N.D., D.C., were also recommending a focus on the out breath as a key to their holistic approaches to treating asthma. Both of these men had written books on holistic approaches to treating asthma after having having suffered severe asthma since childhood. Dr. Firshein, author of *Reversing Asthma,* realized the benefits of this type of breathing while he was hospitalized during a potentially life threatening episode of asthma. Somehow it occurred to him to breathe in for seven counts of his heartbeat while breathing out for a count of nine. His recovery was much faster than expected. Since then he has developed and incorporated breathing techniques into his practice and classes with great success. Dr. Roberts, having experienced severe asthma from the age of eight, also learned to breathe more effectively on his own. His book, *Asthma: An Alternative Approach,* teaches breathing exercises similar to what we are presenting here, while mentioning the Buteyko method. In one study on "Complementary Therapies for Asthma" performed in the United Kingdom, breathing techniques were used by 44 percent of the severe asthmatics, far more than any other modality. The majority found them to be moderately useful.

As traumatic as the experience of asthma is, it can become an invitation "you can't refuse," to learn how to intervene and consciously take control of breathing effectively. You can choose to see the asthmatic attacks as warnings your body is sending you, and use the experience as an opportunity to begin practicing more conscious and effective breathing—an act of loving your lungs. Breathing this way can help to break the cycle of panic and shortness of breath that builds up during an asthma attack. Empowered with these new techniques, you can begin challenging yourself to see if you can prevent attacks and/or lessen the intensity of an attack while in the midst of one. As your lungs become better conditioned, it becomes easier to practice. Conscious breathing allows you to be much more in control and no longer a victim.

By learning to be more aware of your breathing patterns and applying a time-honored blend of traditional yogic techniques with newer, clinically proven methods, you will be able to lessen the frequency, duration, and intensity of asthma attacks. Used in conjunction with the entire Asthma Survival Program, it is also possible to eliminate asthma altogether. In spite of the fact that the National Lung Association acknowledges the therapeutic benefits of breathing exercises for people with asthma, there are far too few physicians actually recommending or teaching them. Dr. Nelson and I, along with many of our holistic physician colleagues, recommend them as a *primary* therapy.

In this chapter we will coach you on a beginning level of breathing exercises. At the end of this section we will direct you to resources for more advanced techniques. Consider this as the first step in putting your lungs into "breathing training camp" in order to condition them for consistently better function. The breathing techniques are based on the fact that people with asthma need to create a better balance of oxygen and carbon dioxide, better overall lung fitness, less muscular tension, a sense of calmness, and a stronger feeling of control. The exercises help to strengthen peripheral and accessory breathing muscles that assist the lungs, thereby relieving the workload of the diaphragm. There is an estimated 20 percent of unused lung capacity at any given time. When your lungs are trained to do so, you can draw on this reserve during times of respiratory distress.

Most people with asthma have a heightened state of chronic muscle tension combined with exhaustion. This is because there is a long-term imbalance in the sympathetic and parasympathetic branches of the nervous system. The parasympathetic branch is like a "brake," creating relaxation, full and easy breathing, sleep, and good digestion. The sympathetic branch acts as the "accelerator." It rouses us to action and puts us into the "fight-or-flight" stress response when we perceive a threat. During the fight-or-flight response, adrenaline is released and breathing becomes shallow and rapid, heart rate and blood pressure go up, and muscles become tense in preparation for action. Being an asthmatic can potentially lead to a perpetual condition of fight-or-flight breathing—a state of stressful, excessive sympathetic nervous function, which eventually exhausts the lungs and the adrenal glands. This usually leads to a greater dependency on medication to regulate breathing. This state of sympathetic excess causes a form of chronic hyperventilation, or overbreathing, and leads to a constant state of hypoxia, or low oxygen in the bloodstream. Hypoxia, in turn, can increase anxiety and fatigue, which can significantly worsen the asthmatic condition.

The Asthma Survival approach to effective breathing techniques synthesizes the principles we have just discussed and starts you on five of the most important exercises. Remember to begin slowly, listen to your body's feedback, and above all, practice at least 3 times daily for 5 to 10 minutes each time *while you are well and asthma-free*. (Many patients choose to practice for a few minutes every hour. This is even more effective.) If for any reason you feel light-headed or out of breath, just take a minute or two to breathe normally and relax. Then try resuming the exercise again. If your sinuses are congested, then I recommend that you steam and do nasal irrigation prior to the exercises to open the nasal passages (see pages 97–102). If at all possible, try to perform these exercises in a clean-air environment.

1. *Basic belly (or abdominal) breathing.* Begin by lying on your back with your knees up and your legs slightly apart. Get comfortable and at first just notice your breathing without trying to do anything. Relax and feel yourself "sinking" into the floor. Then place your open hands around your lower rib cage, with your palms at the lower part of your ribs and your fingertips touching at your belly button. Feel the lower parts of your ribs expand and your belly rise up easily and smoothly as you breathe in through your nose. Now breathe out long and slow through your nose or mouth as you feel your belly sink. When breathing out through your mouth, keep your lips close together, firmly pushing the air out. Try not to engage your shoulders or upper chest in the breathing effort. See if you can comfortably breath out for 4 to 5 seconds or more and in for 1 to 3 seconds. Go slowly, don't overbreathe, and let the breath out long and slow while you relax and sink deeper into the floor. The out breath will relax you more and more. Breathing out will create air hunger and naturally encourage an inhalation. Let the in breath be slow, smooth, and through the nose. Feel the inhale deep in the back of your throat, but *do not take in a forced, large inhalation.* Remember that you want to emphasize a complete out breath. Try working toward breathing out for 8 to 12 seconds and in for 2 to 4. To feel your belly muscles even more, you may want to place a book or something that has some added weight on your abdomen for kinesthetic feedback. Once you are comfortable with this exercise, add a variation: At the end of the outbreath, try to hum, or add an *mmmm* or *nnnnn* sound to expel even more residual air. Stop, of course, if this aggravates wheezing.

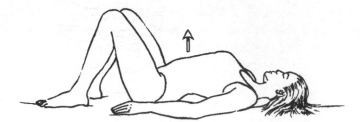

FIGURE 4.2

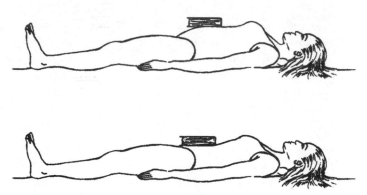

FIGURE 4.3

2. *Belly Breathing while seated.* Use the same instructions as above, but while sitting in a chair. Keep your hands wrapped around your lower ribs to get a good feel of the muscular action. This is good to do at the office, in class, even in traffic—but keep both hands on the wheel!
3. *Belly breathing while walking.* While you are well and relatively asthma-free, try walking for 5 to 15 minutes at a time, 1 to 3 times daily. Start slowly and remember to focus on the out breath, starting with a count of 4 out and 2 in. Try adding 2 counts on the out breath over time but keeping the in breath shorter. The basic rule is that the exhalation should be at least two times longer than the in-

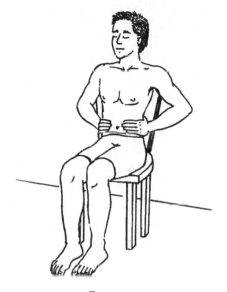

FIGURE 4.4

halation. Over a period of weeks or months, depending on your condition, try building the count on the out breath to more than 10. Try adding a light hissing or whooshing sound from your lips while exhaling once you are tolerating the exercise well. Be patient and persistent. This helps condition the lungs for longer endurance and aerobic conditioning. Once you are tolerating this exercise well, you may want to try it on a mini-trampoline, also called a rebounder, while gently bouncing. The bouncing motion promotes lymphatic circulation and oxygenation.

4. *Belly breathing while lying over the back of an easy chair.* Best done by children with asthma. (*Caution:* Those who are elderly, or have high blood pressure, vertigo or inner-ear problems, active sinus or respiratory infection, headaches, or neck and back disorders, should NOT do this.) Kneel on a well-padded easy chair, bending over the back of the chair at the waist and letting the head and arms hang free. Practice the belly breathing. This position promotes exhalation. Perform the exercise only for 1 to 5 minutes at a time.

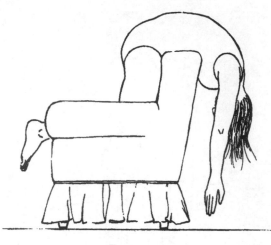

FIGURE 4.5

5. *Belly Breathing while in the midst of an asthma attack.* If in bed, lie on your side in a fetal position, which will promote relaxation of your rib cage. Perform regular belly breathing and try to relax into sleep.

Another natural postural position to assume at the onset of an attack is kneeling on a comfortable floor, sitting on your feet, folding your arms on a low table or seat, with your head resting on your arms. Begin breathing very gently out as far as possible without triggering wheezing. It may take 10 to 20 minutes of practicing the belly breathing before you can get relief. Keep relaxing and letting go of tension in your upper chest, shoulders, and neck. Let the diaphragm do most of the work. If your attack isn't relieved in short order, take the remedies prescribed to you and continue the breathing—long, slow and out, easily in through the nose.

Conditioned belly breathing can profoundly alter the course of your asthma and hasten your ability to not only survive, but to thrive with much more energy, greater immunity, and aliveness!

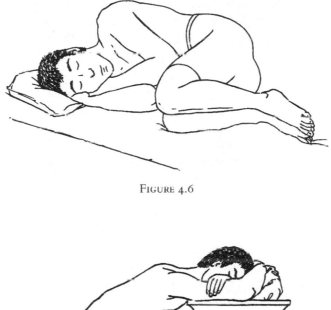

FIGURE 4.6

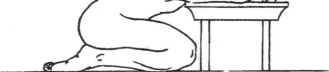

FIGURE 4.7

2. WATER, MOISTURE, AND NASAL HYGIENE

Next to oxygen, *water* is our most essential nutrient, and drinking enough water to satisfy your body's needs may be the simplest, least expensive (other than abdominal breathing) self-help measure you can adopt to maintain your overall good health, in addition to the health of your mucous membranes.

Our adult bodies are 60 to 70 percent water (an infant's body is about 80 percent), and water is the medium through which every bodily function occurs. It is the basis of all body fluids, including blood, digestive juices, urine, lymph, and perspiration, which explains why we would die within a few days without water.

Water is vital to metabolism and digestion and helps prevent both constipation and diarrhea. It is also critical to healthy nerve impulse conduction and brain function. Some of water's other vital functions in the body are:

- Enhancing oxygen uptake into the bloodstream. (The surface of the lungs must be moistened with water to facilitate oxygen intake and the excretion of carbon dioxide.)
- Maintaining a high urine volume, helping to prevent kidney stones and urinary tract infections
- Regulating body temperature through perspiration
- Maintaining and increasing the health of the skin
- Maintaining adequate fluid for the lubrication of the joints and enhancing muscular function, particularly during and after exercise or other strenuous activity
- Moistening the mucous membranes of the respiratory tract, which in turn increases resistance to infection and thins the mucus, allowing it to drain more easily

Because water is so important to our health, all of us need to make a conscious effort to stay well hydrated, since most of us lose water faster than we replace it. For example, we lose one pint of water each day simply through exhalation. We also lose the same amount through perspiration, as well as three additional pints per day through urination and defecation. Exercise and heat exposure, especially in a dry climate, also increase water loss in the body. The percentage of body water content also decreases with age. All told, on average, each of us loses two and a half quarts of water (80 ounces) per day under normal conditions. Therefore, it is essential that the same amount or more be replenished daily.

Unfortunately, most Americans don't come close to consuming that much water per day. As a result, many of us are chronically dehydrated. When we think of dehydration, we may envision a lost soul in the desert, dying of thirst. However, most conditions of dehydration are not that dramatic, so that dehydration all too often is unsuspected and therefore undiagnosed. Meanwhile, its insidious effects can wreak havoc on our health by chronically impacting every one of our bodily functions. The results are:

- Reduced blood volume, with less oxygen and nutrients provided to all muscles and organs
- Reduced brain size and impaired neuromuscular coordination, concentration, and thinking
- Excess body fat
- Poor muscle tone and size
- Impaired digestive function and constipation
- Increased toxicity in the body
- Joint and muscle pain
- Water retention (edema), which can result in a state of being overweight and also impede weight loss
- Hyperconcentration of blood with increased viscosity, leading to higher risk of heart attack

Even though you may not be feeling thirsty, you may nonetheless be one of the millions of Americans who are chronically dehydrated. And if you have asthma, it may be especially harmful. Dehydration can cause your body to produce histamine (a substance that can cause inflammation of the mucous membrane and trigger asthma) in an effort to prevent water loss through the lungs. Observation of your urine is one simple way to determine if you are. If your urine is heavy, cloudy, and deep yellow, orange, or brown in tint, it's more than likely that you are dehydrated. The urine of a properly hydrated body tends to be light and nearly clear in color, similar in appearance to unsweetened lemonade. As your water intake approaches your daily need for it, you will notice the appearance of your urine changing accordingly. (Remember that B vitamins will also turn urine a dark yellow.)

Because dehydration is so deceptive—it can occur without

symptoms of thirst—in general, we need to drink more water than our thirst calls for. This does not mean coffee, soft drinks, or alcohol, all of which contribute further to dehydration. Even processed fruit juices and milk are not healthy substitutes for water, because of the sugar and possible pesticides in the former and the hormones and antibiotics in the latter.

The exact amount of water a person needs depends on a number of individual factors, such as body weight, diet, metabolic rate, climate, level of physical activity, and stress factors. Some health professionals recommend that we all drink eight 8-ounce glasses of water a day. A more accurate rule of thumb is to drink half an ounce of water per pound of body weight if you are a healthy but sedentary adult, and to increase that amount to two-thirds of an ounce per pound if you are an active exerciser. This means that a healthy, sedentary adult weighing 160 pounds should drink about ten 8-ounce glasses of water per day, while an active exerciser should drink thirteen to fourteen 8-ounce glasses. If your diet is particularly high in fresh fruits and vegetables, your daily water intake needs may be less, since these foods are 85 to 90 percent water in content and can help restore lost fluids. Herbal teas, natural fruit juices (without sugar added and diluted 50 percent with water), and soups that are sugarless and low in salt (the thinner the better) are also acceptable substitutes for drinking water.

Nearly as important as the amount of water you drink is the *quality* of your water. Simply put, if you aren't drinking filtered water, then your body is forced to become the filter. Still, it's impossible to generalize about whether you should drink tap, bottled, or filtered water. (Distilled water is not recommended for drinking, because it lacks necessary minerals and can also leach them from your body.) In some communities, water purity is so high that it requires no treatment, while other water sources are contaminated with high concentrations of lead and radon, the two worst contaminants.

Another issue related to our drinking water is chlorination. Since chlorine was first introduced into America's drinking water supply in 1908, it has eliminated epidemics of cholera, dysentery, and typhoid. Multiple studies, however, now suggest an association between chlorine and increased free-radical production, which can lead to a higher incidence of cancer. On the positive side, chlorine is effective in eliminating most microorganisms from drinking water. (One notable exception is the parasite Cryptosporidium, which is resistant to chlorine.)

Unless you live in one of the communities that supply pure water, drinking tap water is not recommended, especially since the majority of health-related risks present in drinking water occur from contamination that is added *after* the water leaves the treatment and distribution plant. This includes pipes that run from municipal systems into your home, lead-soldered copper pipes, and fixtures that contain lead and may leach lead or other toxic metals (such as cadmium, mercury, and cobalt) into your tap water. Therefore, if you drink tap water, it would be a good idea to have the water from your tap tested, regardless of the claims from your local water utility. You can get started by calling your local health department for a referral for testing.

Because of the growing concerns regarding tap water, increasing numbers of Americans now choose bottled water for drinking and cooking purposes. This can not only prove to be expensive, but also may not be as safe as you think. Regulations mandated for the bottled-water industry are similar to those followed by the public water treatment industry and currently do not include required testing for Cryptosporidium and many other contaminants. Moreover, 25 percent of bottled water sold in this country comes from filtered municipal water that is then treated. For this reason, perhaps the healthiest choice regarding your drinking water is to invest in a water filter. Reverse-osmosis filters appear to be the most effective home water-filtering systems presently available. But there are also some distillation and carbon filters that are able to reduce lead in water significantly. There are carafe-style filters for the kitchen faucet that cost about $25, under-the-sink models for $400, and units that purify the water as it enters the house. These can cost as much as $1,250.

Since it is impossible to always know for certain whether what we drink or eat is completely safe, do the best you can. To get in the habit of drinking enough water, spread your intake throughout the day (drinking very little after dinner), and don't drink more than four 8-ounce glasses in any one-hour period. It's also best to drink between meals so as not to interfere with your body's digestive process. Make your water drinking convenient; keep a container of water at hand, in your car, or at your desk, and don't wait until you feel thirsty to start drinking. Most important, be sure that there's always a bathroom nearby. The belief that you can stretch your bladder is a myth.

Drinking good-quality water and in the appropriate amounts is recommended for anyone interested in experiencing optimal health. However, the remainder of this section is more directed at the individual who is treating or preventing the most common respiratory conditions—asthma, sinusitis, and allergies. *Moisture* can help to thin the thick mucus filling the bronchioles of asthmatics, in addition to emptying a sick sinus of its thick, infected mucus. In doing so it helps to restore normal cilial function and relieve wheezing, nasal and head congestion, headache, sinus pain, and sore throat. Warm, moist air is best, and the easiest place to get it is in the bathroom. Steamers can now be installed in showers, or simply close any doors and windows and turn the shower on hot to create steam. You then have the choice of either getting in the shower—after adjusting the temperature, of course—or just sitting and relaxing in the steam until you run out of hot water. Make a conscious effort to breathe through your nose. Hot towels applied over the face can also be helpful for relieving the symptoms of sinusitis.

As most of us do not have an endless supply of hot water or steamers, making a steam room of the bathroom can be done only two or three times a day. What about the rest of the time? If you are staying home from work, your best source of moist air is a humidifier placed by your bed, with the bedroom door and windows closed (see page 80). Whatever your choice of humidifier, be sure the reservoir tank opening is large enough to allow for cleaning. Wipe and cleanse the tank at least weekly with vinegar water; otherwise it becomes a breeding ground for molds, which are becoming a more common cause of asthma and chronic sinusitis. If you're treating or preventing a sinus infection or asthma, the humidifier should be used every night while you sleep. It's also a good idea to fill it and turn it on as soon as you come home from work so your bedroom will be warm and moist by the time you're ready for bed. The moisture is very helpful in relieving the infection's cough and sore throat during the night. To minimize mold, I would empty the humidifier every morning and allow it to dry out. Be aware that there are a few asthmatics who feel worse with too much humidity. Try to adjust the moisture level to suit your individual needs, but understand that the mucous membranes are generally healthier with at least 35 percent relative humidity.

Another device I've been using preventively on myself and recommending to patients as part of their asthma and/or sinus treatment program is the Steam Inhaler (see Figure 4.8). It's extremely effective for thinning and loosening the thick infected

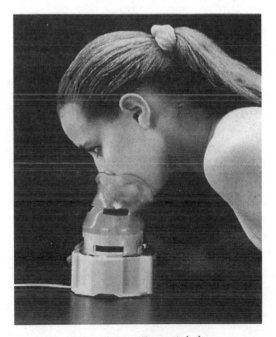

FIGURE 4.8 *Steam inhaler*

or non-infected mucus stuck in the sinuses and bronchioles, and can be quite soothing to dry and irritated mucous membranes while also relieving sinus headaches. There is evidence that steam also helps to open your airway and can act as a decongestant and bronchodilator. A few drops or a spray of medicinal eucalyptus oil added to the unit while you are steaming enhances its therapeutic effect. I've also added a few drops of the Sinus Survival Spray to the Inhaler. (If you are treating a sinus infection, you can add a drop or two of tea tree oil, a powerful anti-infective herb.) To benefit the entire mucous membrane while steaming, alternate inhaling through your nose (upper respiratory tract) and your mouth (lower respiratory tract—lungs). If used just prior to nasal irrigation, a procedure that I'm about to explain, it will greatly increase the benefit of the irrigation. The Steam Inhaler I use is made by Kaz, costs about $50, but unfortunately is no longer readily available. Complete information on where to obtain any of the products I mention is listed in the Product Index at the end of the book.

Assuming your environment is relatively dry, as indoor air tends to be during the winter months in most parts of the United States, you can also provide moisture with a saltwater (also called *saline*) *nasal spray*. There are several commercial products available in pharmacies. However, you can make your own saline spray by mixing one quarter to one half of a teaspoon of non-iodized table salt and a pinch of baking soda in an 8-ounce cup of lukewarm bottled water (without chlorine) and dispensing it from a spray bottle. You can use sea salt without iodine. Spray into each nostril while closing off the other nostril and simultaneously inhaling. This is nonaddictive and can be done as often as you like throughout the day. It has no negative side effects, except for the curious looks you will get from those wanting to know what you are spraying in your nose.

The Sinus Survival Spray, a botanical saline nasal mist, has been a highly effective addition to the Sinus Survival Program. Formulated by Dr. Steve Morris, a naturopathic physician from Mukilteo, Washington, and myself, we have been using it on ourselves and recommending it to our patients for more than seven years, with excellent results. In addition to saline, which makes up the bulk of the spray, the ingredients include:

- Goldenseal: acts as an antibacterial, antifungal, and anti-inflammatory
- Selenium: a powerful antioxidant with anti-allergic and anti-inflammatory capability
- Aloe vera: has antifungal properties and relieves irritation
- Grapefruit-seed extract: an excellent antifungal

The first three ingredients are all soothing and healing to the nasal mucous membranes. The selenium has allowed the product to be used as part of the allergy treatment program as well as for sinusitis. I've even used this spray as an eyedrop and found it quite soothing for dry and irritated eyes caused by air pollution and arid conditions. When the spray bottle is turned upside down, it can function as an eyedropper. The Sinus Survival Spray is available in many health food stores and can also be obtained through Sinus Survival Products.

An even more effective way of moisturizing is *saline irrigation.* This procedure can result in dramatic relief from pain by reducing swelling in the nasal passages, causing a reduction of pressure in the sinus, as well as helping to empty the sinus of its infected mucus. Saltwater sprays also irrigate—that is, wash out—some mucus, bacteria, and dust particles, while reducing swelling. However, they don't do it as well as the following irrigation methods. Throughout the past decade I've heard many people comment that nasal irrigation, using any of the first three techniques described below, has been the *single most helpful component* of the entire Sinus Survival Program. For anyone with asthma who also suffers with sinusitis, this procedure would be an essential part of their Asthma Survival Program. Irrigation should be done three to four times a day for acute sinusitis and once or twice for a milder chronic condition. Many former sinus sufferers continue to irrigate daily on a preventive basis, even after curing their chronic sinusitis.

Mix the saline solution for irrigation fresh each day in one cup of lukewarm bottled water. Add one quarter to one half of a teaspoon of non-iodized table salt or sea salt and a tiny pinch of baking soda, thus making the solution close to normal body-fluid salinity and pH. Irrigating with plain water is usually somewhat uncomfortable. Use the full cup of saline solution for each irrigation (one-half cup for each nostril). Lean over the sink, with the head rotated so that the nostril to be irrigated is directly above the other nostril, while using one of the following methods. Always blow your nose *very gently* after irrigating.

Method 1 For the past seven years I have been recommending the use of the Neti Pot, and more recently SinuCleanse, for nasal irrigation. "Neti Pot" is a small porcelain pot with a narrow spout (SinuCleanse is plastic with a very similar shape and size). This is probably the most gentle and convenient method for irrigation. Because of this, people with chronic sinusitis are much more apt to use this method on a regular basis, both therapeutically in treating an infection and preventively. SinuCleanse is sold with packets of hypertonic saline to mix with water, making this method even more convenient. The Neti Pot is made by the Himalayan Institute in Honesdale, Pennsylvania, and is available in many health food stores. SinuCleanse is available through Sinus Survival Products.

Method 2 Use an angled nasal irrigator attachment (the Grossan nasal irrigator is available at some pharmacies) on a Water Pik appliance. Set the Water Pik at the *lowest* possible pressure and insert the irrigator tip just inside one nostril, pinching your nostril to form a seal. Irrigate with your mouth open, allowing the fluid to drain out either your mouth or nose. Repeat the procedure in the other nostril. The pulsations of the Water Pik makes this perhaps the most effective method for irrigation. However, it is also the most expensive.

Method 3 Completely fill a large, all-rubber ear syringe (available at most pharmacies) with saline solution. Lean over the sink and insert the syringe tip just inside one nostril, so that it forms a comfortable seal. *Gently* squeeze and release the bulb several times to swish the solution around the inside of your nose. The solution will run out both nostrils and may also run out of your mouth. Repeat this for each nostril until one cup of saline solution is used, or until the solution is clear.

Method 4 For very small children, irrigate with ten to twenty drops of saline solution per nostril from an eyedropper.

If you are using a decongestant nasal spray or a corticosteroid nasal spray, use them only *after* the saltwater nasal irrigations.

These methods obviously require more effort than the saline nasal sprays, but many patients comment on how much more helpful it is.

Another solution that has been effective in irrigation is called Alkalol. It is a mucus solvent and cleaner, and can be used with the saline solution in a 1:1 ratio (one half saline, one half Alka lol) with all of the methods previously mentioned. You will probably have to ask your pharmacist to order it for you, as it is not usually available, but Alkalol is very inexpensive.

Water, moisture, and nasal hygiene—that is, saline spray, steam, and irrigation—can also help to relieve the symptoms of dry, crusted nasal membranes that are common with chronic sinusitis and often prone to nosebleeds. You can apply Neosporin ointment or even better Ponaris nasal emollient (ask your pharmacist to order it) to the nasal membranes twice daily with a Q-Tip or your little finger.

The beneficial effects of nasal irrigation for chronic sinusitis are obvious to anyone with this condition who has irrigated regularly. However, it was not until a Spanish physician, Jose Luis Subiza, M.D., performed a recent study in Madrid using the Grossan nasal irrigator with allergy sufferers that the benefits of irrigation for allergies was documented. They found that irrigating the nose with saline three times a day during the grass pollen season (May to July) significantly reduced the allergic response to grass. This finding also supports the critical role of the nasal mucous membrane in the allergic response. And it reinforces the primary objective of the Sinus and Asthma Survival Program: *to heal the mucous membranes!*

CANDIDA AND FUNGUS

On the morning of December 28, 2000, I was greeted with the *Denver Post*'s front-page headline article: "Antibiotics Spawn More 'Superbugs'—As overuse continues, drug-resistant bacteria on rise." My first reaction was "So what else is new." The threat of drug-resistant bacteria has been recognized for more than a decade, but what three new studies were reporting is that the problem has steadily worsened despite warnings from scientists that bacteria are adapting to the excessive use of antibiotics by evolving into hard-to-kill "superbugs." Researchers estimate that half of all antibiotics prescribed by doctors are unnecessary, given to patients with viral infections or other ailments that the drugs will not fight. With pneumococcal infections (from a bacterium that commonly causes pneumonia, ear infections, and meningitis), the proportion of these caused by strains of pneumococcal bacteria that were resistant to three classes of antibiotics had risen from 9 percent in 1995 to 14 percent in 1998; the proportion resistant to penicillin had risen from 21 to 25 percent. In children under 5, the rate of penicillin resistance was 32 percent. Dr. Cynthia Whitney, a medical epidemiologist who directed one of the new studies, which appeared in both the *New England Journal of Medicine* and the *Journal of the American Medical Association,* attributed the increase to "survival of the fittest," in which bacteria with natural resistance to a given antibiotic manage to withstand treatment and multiply. If the same antibiotic is given again, the process repeats itself. Gradually, resistant bacteria predominate, making the antibiotic less and less effective.

From my own clinical observations, I believe that the overuse of antibiotics has contributed to a gradual weakening and dysfunction of the immune system that facilitates the survival and growth of these supergerms, in addition to causing an over-growth of yeast organisms, or candidiasis. In fact, a 1999 study performed in New Zealand at the Wellington School of Medicine, found that antibiotic use in infancy may be associated with a significantly increased risk of developing asthma.

In at least two-thirds of asthmatics there is a history of recurrent sinusitis. Almost every one of these sinus infections is treated with broad-spectrum antibiotics. In the first Sinus Survival Study, completed in March 2000, the ten participants each had moderate to severe chronic sinusitis that had not responded to conventional treatment—antibiotics and, in several instances, surgery. All of them scored above 180 on the Candida Questionnaire (page 115), four had asthma besides the sinusitis, and each was treated with the antifungal (candida is a type of fungus) drug Diflucan 200 mg/day for six weeks in addition to the entire Sinus Survival Program. Following this course of treatment, nine of the ten participants experienced a dramatic improvement in their sinus symptoms (many were feeling better than they had in years), while three of the four asthmatics reported similar results with their asthma—much less difficulty breathing, along with a significant reduction in their need for their inhalers. The one person who did not improve was the most severely ill. During the course of the Diflucan, he developed a sinus infection that triggered a flare-up of his asthma and was prescribed antibiotics and prednisone. These medications negated the therapeutic effect of the Diflucan. This study provides evidence supporting the findings of the 1999 Mayo Clinic study. They reported that *an immune system response to fungus rather than bacterial infection is the cause of most cases of chronic sinusitis.* The investigators reached this conclusion after studying 210 patients with chronic sinusitis and discovered 40 different kinds of fungus, including candida, in the mucus of 96 percent of them. In a control group of normal healthy volunteers they found very similar organisms. They therefore concluded that the immune system response to these fungi in patients with chronic sinusitis is markedly different than in healthy people, and this unusual immune reaction is responsible for the chronic inflammation,

pain, and swelling of the mucous membrane associated with sinusitis. I believe that a similar immune dysfunction triggered by
fungal organisms and a yeast overgrowth is responsible for many
cases of moderate and severe asthma. There was, in fact, another
study published in 1999 in the *Journal of Allergy and Clinical Immunology* that lends more support to the fungus–asthma connection. Eleven patients with adult-onset moderate or severe
asthma plus fungal skin infections were treated with Diflucan
100 mg daily for five months. This treatment resulted in marked
improvement of their symptoms, a significant increase in pulmonary function, a dramatic decrease in hospitalizations, emergency room visits, and medication (oral steroids) requirements.
The Asthma Survival Program recognizes the potential causal
link between fungus/candida and asthma and includes this as a
primary aspect of asthma treatment. Since diet comprises the
bulk of the treatment for candida, the discussion of this subject
is included in the "Candida Treatment" section on page 121.

Yeast is an integral part of life. It is a hardy fungus found in
food, air, and on the exposed surfaces of most objects. There are
more than 250 species of yeast organisms, and more than 150 of
them can be found as harmless parasites in the human body. The
most prevalent type of yeast found in and on our bodies is *Candida albicans.* It is an innocuous single-cell fungus and a normal
inhabitant of our intestines, mouth, nose, sinuses, lungs, and
vagina. Although not well documented, it is believed that its
only function is to help absorb the B vitamins.

Candida is kept under control by the good bacteria that also
make their home in the human gastrointestinal, respiratory, and
genital tracts. A large percentage of the millions of these
friendly bacteria are lactobacillus and bifidus. Similar to the bacteria in yogurt or in raw fermented foods, the lactobacilli make
enzymes and vitamins, help fight undesirable bacteria, and lower
cholesterol levels. While assisting us in keeping our bowel function and digestion normal, these friendly bacteria, also referred
to as acidophilus bacteria, regard candida as their food. Since
they are the chief "predator" of candida, they are critical to
maintaining a "balance of nature" in our intestines. As long as

this homeostatic relationship is maintained, candida poses no problem. However, to an increasing extent, massive overgrowth of candida is resulting in a condition medically known as candidiasis, candida-related complex, or candida toxicity syndrome. *The most frequent cause of this imbalance is the recurrent or extended use of antibiotics,* which kill the "good" bacteria and, hopefully, those causing the infection for which the antibiotic is being taken. The more broad-spectrum the antibiotic, the broader the range of bacteria it will eliminate, therefore killing more of the lactobacilli. Millions of women are familiar with vaginal yeast infections, which develop when, or just after, using antibiotics. What I have repeatedly observed in my practice is that the vast majority of people with both chronic sinusitis and asthma, who have taken three or more ten-day to two-week courses of antibiotics within a six-month period, probably have some degree of candidiasis. Since most antibiotics are given by mouth, the friendly bacteria of the intestines are particularly vulnerable to these medications.

Hormones, especially progesterone, and birth control pills can also contribute to causing candidiasis, which is why the overgrowth of candida is more prevalent in women than in men, children, or nonmenstruating women. Progesterone, found in most birth control pills and also secreted at high levels during the ten to fourteen days prior to menstruation, has been shown to stimulate the growth of candida. The combination of high progesterone levels just prior to menstruation and an existing excess of candida can contribute to particularly severe symptoms of PMS (premenstrual syndrome). As you will see in Table 4.8 on page 165, many of the symptoms of candidiasis are also present with PMS. Pregnancy is also favorable for candida, since it is accompanied by continuous high levels of progesterone.

Anything that weakens the immune system can contribute to yeast overgrowth or help to trigger the immune response to candida and fungi observed in the Mayo Clinic study. Cortisone medications, such as prednisone and prednisolone, often used in treating asthma, are well-known immune system suppressants. They, too, have the potential for stimulating candidiasis, and can actually aggravate the disease the cortisone was treating. Chemotherapy and radiation treatments given to cancer patients can also weaken immunity and open the door to candida.

Any medication that can potentially cause gastrointestinal ulcerations or inflammation and weaken the lining of the gut can allow candida to gain a stronger and deeper foothold. These drugs may include aspirin, cortisone, and nonsteroidal anti-inflammatories such as Feldene, Naprosyn, Anaprox, Motrin, Advil, and Nuprin. Medicines given to ulcer patients, such as Tagamet and Zantac, can reduce acidity and raise pH levels high enough for yeast to grow. Candida thrive in a pH of 4 to 5, and normal stomach acidity is 2 to 3.

Environmental toxins and chemicals such as pesticides, herbicides, solvents, paints, formaldehyde, pentachlorophenol, combustion products of natural gas and coal (sulfur and nitrous oxide), petrochemicals (exhausts), and heavy metals such as lead, cadmium, arsenic, mercury, aluminum, and nickel can also weaken the immune system. People with occupational exposure to these substances are at highest risk for candidiasis, but most of us in urban America live in such a toxic environment that we are all probably receiving significant exposure.

Other conditions that can cause immune dysfunction and can thereby potentially allow yeast overgrowth to occur are: allergies to inhalants, foods, or chemicals; viral infections such as Epstein-Barr virus (EBV), cytomegalovirus (CMV), human immunodeficiency virus (HIV), chronic or recurring flu illnesses; intestinal parasitic infections brought on by amoeba, giardia, or ascaris; hypothyroidism; nutrient deficiencies due to a poor diet or digestive problems (hydrochloric acid, pancreatic enzymes, and bile); major surgery; and emotional stress. The more severe the condition, the greater the potential for candidiasis.

Once the scale has been tipped and the overgrowth begins, it is fueled by the staple of the typical American diet—sugar. Like most of us, yeast consider sugar to be their favorite food. While candida thrive on it, sugar weakens our immune system. It decreases the ability of white blood cells, phagocytes in particular, to engulf unwanted organisms. It is therefore no surprise that diabetes, a chronic condition of high blood sugar, is also a major predisposing factor to candidiasis.

Obviously, there are a multitude of causes that can contribute to creating the condition of candidiasis and/or trigger the unusual immune response to fungi. In most instances it is the combination of several factors occurring simultaneously that actually precipitates the overgrowth of yeast and the atypical immune reaction. In patients with both asthma and chronic sinusitis, the primary causes are most often: (1) repeated broad-spectrum antibiotics along with, (2) a sugar-filled diet, and (3) significant emotional stress. As a general rule in medicine, as in life, there is rarely just one cause for anything. However, in my experience, *in almost every instance of a particularly resistant case of chronic sinusitis along with moderate to severe asthma, candida is a primary cause.*

Symptoms of Candida

Once the overgrowth occurs, the yeast invade the tissues of the gastrointestinal tract by growing in a plantlike form and sending roots into the walls of the small intestine. These roots can eventually bore holes in the intestinal wall, causing a condition known as "leaky gut syndrome." This means that the damage to the wall is allowing candida, bacteria, food, pollen, environmental pollutants, and other material to enter the bloodstream. It's almost as if your intestine has become a superabsorbent sponge. Candida often travel through the rectum and anus to the vagina and urinary tract and can subsequently enter the bloodstream via this more indirect route. Candida are then carried throughout the body and take up residence in those parts of the body with the most favorable environment for their growth—moist mucous membranes, especially those of the sinuses and lungs. In whatever tissue the candida have colonized, they cause inflammation and subsequent physical discomfort, such as sinus pain, wheezing, muscle aches, joint pain, and itchy anus or vagina. There is still some controversy surrounding this point: Are the candida organisms themselves traveling through the bloodstream and causing these symptoms throughout the body,

Table 4.1

Factors Tipping the Balance in Favor of Yeast

Antibiotics, primarily from medicines, also from commercial meats
and poultry
Birth control pills
Pregnancy
Cortisone and other immunosuppressant drugs
Sugar
Alcohol
Typical American diet (high fat, high sugar, nutrient-poor)
Environmental chemicals
Chemotherapy and radiation
Free radicals
Food and other allergies
Malabsorption of nutrients
Deficiencies of hydrochloric acid, pancreatic enzymes, and bile
Undiagnosed hypothyroidism
Chronic viral infections
Occult parasitic infections, especially giardia and amoeba
Diabetes
Anti-inflammatory and other medications that produce gastrointesti-
nal ulcerations
Acid antagonists (ulcer medications)
Major surgery
Physical trauma
Emotional trauma
Poor coping mechanisms to life's stresses
Diarrhea
Adrenal dysfunction—increased cortisol and decreased DHEA

Reprinted with permission from *Optimal Wellness* by Ralph T. Golan, M.D.,
Ballantine Books, 1995.

or is it the toxins that have been released from candida? The predominant belief currently is that it is most likely the toxins, since those people with detectable candida in the bloodstream are *dying*. This includes patients with AIDS, cancer, and other degenerative conditions where the mucous barrier/immunity is so low that yeast organisms have crossed over into the bloodstream. As a result of widespread inflammation in the small bowel from the direct toxicity of candida, symptoms of the gastrointestinal tract are usually noticed first. Due to incomplete digestion and poor absorption of nutrients, these symptoms may include bloating, a feeling of fullness, diarrhea, constipation, alternating diarrhea and constipation, rectal itching, gas, and cramping. If the inflammation is severe and/or long-standing, it may be another contributing factor to causing leaky gut syndrome. As a result of this condition, large undigested particles of food, especially proteins, pass into the bloodstream and trigger multiple food allergies and sensitivities.

But the greatest health risks presented by candida result from the toxins they release (seventy-nine different ones have been identified), which can damage tissues directly or circulate throughout the bloodstream and cause problems in distant organs. These toxins can also significantly weaken the immune system by inhibiting the function of suppressor T-cells. These white blood cells, a type of lymphocyte, are responsible for modulating antibody production. When they are not working, there is a resulting excess of antibodies. The combination of this overabundance of antibodies along with the absorption of incompletely digested protein helps to explain the exaggerated sensitivities and *multiple adult-onset allergies,* both airborne and food, experienced by many people suffering "systemic" (whole body) candidiasis. The immune system sees the protein particles as antigens or foreign invaders of the body and initiates a powerful "attack," resulting in an allergic reaction.

A yeast-impaired immune system also has less than the normal tolerance for ordinarily safe levels of common chemical odors such as gas and oil fumes, cleaning fluids, chlorine, and perfume. An increasing number of people with candidiasis have become so allergic that almost every odor, all clothing except cotton, almost all foods, or anything in their immediate environment has become a major health problem. This condition has several names: multiple chemical sensitivity, environmental or ecological illness, or the universal reactor phenomenon. The immune system weakened by candida can also produce antibodies to the body's own tissues, especially the ovaries and thyroid, resulting in PMS and hypothyroid symptoms. These symptoms may include fatigue, irritability, sugar craving, headache, depression, and constipation.

One of the major toxins produced by yeast is acetaldehyde. Its multiple effects can be devastating. It is converted by the liver into alcohol, depleting the body of magnesium and potassium, reducing cell energy, and causing symptoms of intoxication—disorientation, dizziness, or mental confusion. The *spaciness* or *mental fog,* as it's often described by patients, is one of the most frequent symptoms of candidiasis. Patients relate a detached state of mind, poor concentration, faulty memory, and difficulty making decisions. The longer this condition persists, the more likely it is that depression will be added to the list of symptoms. The less oxygen in the body, the worse these symptoms are. Exercise, which supplies more oxygen, becomes more difficult to do because of this low-energy state. Energy is also depleted because *acetaldehyde interferes with glucose metabolism—a key component of energy production.* Along with other yeast toxins, *acetaldehyde reduces the absorption of protein and minerals, which in turn diminishes the production of enzymes and hormones needed for energy.* The combination of these multiple factors explains why **excessive fatigue** is the chief complaint of people with candidiasis. It usually comes on gradually but is most noticeable after a night's rest, after eating, and in mid- to late afternoon. When you seek medical attention for extreme fatigue, a physical exam and lab tests will typically be normal. You may even be told, "It's all in your head!" And if you weren't depressed before, you could begin to feel that way now!

The specific organ, tissue, or system damaged by candida will determine which symptoms occur. Table 4.2 is a comprehensive list of the possible symptoms of candidiasis. Many of them have other causes as well. However, if you have several, in addition to a history that is compatible with a yeast overgrowth, you can be relatively certain of the diagnosis.

Diagnosis

The most reliable way to make the diagnosis of candida is by compiling a thorough history and reviewing symptoms. If you are experiencing several of the possible symptoms and have a story compatible with causing candidiasis, there are few laboratory tests that are as dependable as this combination for establishing the diagnosis. However, further confirmation could also be attained through the results of the treatment for yeast or a clinical evaluation by a physician knowledgeable about yeast-related illness. He or she may also employ laboratory techniques such as stool cultures for candida and measurements of antibody levels for candida or candida antigens in the blood (see page 119 for further details). However, while these laboratory exams are useful aids, they should not be solely depended upon to confirm the diagnosis. In other words, the diagnosis is best made by evaluation of a person's history and clinical picture. In his book *The Yeast Connection,* William Crook, M.D., has formalized the symptom and history information into the Candida Questionnaire and Score Sheet, which can be ordered separately from Professional Books, P.O. Box 3494, Jackson, TN 38301. In his book, Dr. Crook says that yeast are especially apt to play a role in causing health problems in patients who:

1. Feel bad "all over," yet the cause can't be identified and treatment of many kinds hasn't helped
2. Have taken prolonged courses of broad-spectrum antibiotics, including tetracycline, ampicillin, amoxicillin, Keflex, Ceclor, Septra, and Bactrim
3. Have consumed diets containing a lot of yeast and sugar
4. Crave sweets
5. Crave other carbohydrates, especially breads and pizza

Table 4.2

Possible Symptoms of Candidiasis

(I have italicized symptoms that are most common.)

Respiratory

Chronic stuffy or runny nose, congested or allergic sinuses, chronic
sneezing or coughing, asthma, shortness of breath/difficulty getting deep breath, recurrent or chronic sore throat, *itchy throat,*
snoring, recurrent colds and flu, *recurrent infections: sinusitis,* tonsilli-
tis, bronchitis, pneumonia, ear infections.

Brain and neurological

Fatigue and lethargy, lack of mental or physical stamina, *depression,*
crying, *mood swings,* anxiety, nervousness, agitation, restlessness,
grumpiness, explosive *irritability,* hostility, suicidal thoughts, *loss of
ability to concentrate,* decreased intellectual functioning, behavior
and learning problems, hyperactivity/poor attention span,
tantrums, *memory impairment,* increasing lack of self-confidence,
impaired ability to reason, *"spacey"* or unreal feeling,
foggy/fuzzy/thick-minded, drunk feeling (without alcohol consumption), *headaches* (all varieties, including migraines), dizziness,
light-headedness, clumsiness/incoordination, shaking, *insomnia,*
"schizophrenia," catatonia, autism, manic-depressive syndrome,
psychosis, multiple sclerosis, myasthenia gravis.

Urogenital

Women: *vaginal itching, burning,* and/or discharge, vulvar itching and
inflammation, vaginal or pelvic pain, painful intercourse, infertility. **Men:** impotence, *recurrent prostatitis* or inflammation of the
prostate. **Both men and women:** *recurrent urethritis/cystitis* (bladder infection), bladder irritations, *burning on urination,* having to
urinate too frequently, bladder "cramping," loss of sex drive.

Skin

Rough, dry, or *scaly skin, acne,* hives, *generalized itching,* eczema,
chronic or recurrent fungal infections of the skin/nails, psoriasis,
easy bruising, recurrent staph infections of the skin, folliculitis,
rosacea, tingling, burning, numbness, and electrical feelings on the
skin.

Ear

Ringing in the ear, stuffed or clogged ear, itching ears, *recurrent ear infections, ear pain, diminished hearing*

Musculoskeletal

Arthritis, arthralgia, *joint pain,* joint stiffness, joint swelling, *muscle pain/aching/*discomfort, muscle weakness, muscle swelling, fatigue.

Gastrointestinal and bowel

Constipation, diarrhea, cramping, excessive gas, *bloating and distention,* intestinal "growling," mucusy or bloody stools, colitis, Crohn's disease, enteritis, irritable bowel syndrome, spastic colon, esophagitis, *indigestion,* heartburn, itchy anus, decreased appetite, oral thrush, canker sore, coated tongue, cracked/fissured tongue, chronic gum inflammation.

Menstrual/female

Premenstrual symptoms: depression, emotional fragility, irritability, *anxiety,* fluid retention (including puffy face and fingers), breast tenderness, abdominal bloating, nausea, headaches, etc. Delayed periods, *irregular periods,* bleeding between periods, scanty or profuse bleeding, passing clots, *painful periods, decreased libido (sexual desire), endometriosis,* infertility, miscarriages, fibrocystic breast disease, under-normal breast development.

Multiple allergies to foods; cravings for sweets, alcohol, bread, and cheese; intolerance or allergy to beverages and foods containing dietary yeasts and molds

Alcoholic beverages, aged cheeses, vinegar, soy sauce, peanuts, bread, brewer's yeast, B vitamins with yeast, mushrooms, bread and other yeast-raised baked items.

Chemical sensitivities

Cigarette smoke, exhaust fumes, perfumes, gasoline odor, new carpets, marking pens, paints, solvents, cleaning agents, etc.

Inhalant allergies

Mold, mildew (overall worsening condition in damp, cold season), "hay fever," dust, etc.

Heart/circulatory system

Rapid heartbeat, mitral valve prolapse, cold hands and feet.

Senses
Disturbances of smell, taste, vision and hearing (i.e., increased sensitivity to noise or light, deafness), salty or metallic taste, *blurred vision, watery eyes.*

Autoimmune
Rheumatoid arthritis, multiple diseases: sclerosis, systemic lupus erythematosus, myasthenia gravis, autoimmune hemolytic anemia, scleroderma, thyroiditis.

Other
Intolerance to heat and cold, hot and cold sweats, underweight, *overweight,* feeling sick all over, fluid retention/edema, anorexia nervosa, tendency to bleed easily/slow clotting.

This list is reprinted from *Optimal Wellness* by Ralph T. Golan, M.D., Ballantine Books, 1995.

6. Notice that sweets make symptoms worse or give a "pickup," followed by a "letdown"
7. Crave alcohol
8. Have taken birth control pills, cortisone, or other corticosteroid drugs
9. Have had multiple pregnancies
10. Have been troubled by recurrent problems related to reproductive organs, including abdominal pain, vaginal infection or discomfort, premenstrual tension, menstrual irregularities, prostatitis, or impotence
11. Are bothered by persistent or recurrent symptoms involving the digestive and nervous systems
12. Have been bothered by athlete's foot, fungus infection of the nails, or jock itch
13. Feel bad on damp days or in moldy places
14. Are made ill when exposed to perfumes, tobacco smoke, and other chemicals

The following is a modification of Dr. Crook's score sheet that can be used to reliably diagnose an overgrowth of candida.

Candida Questionnaire and Score Sheet

This questionnaire is designed for adults and the scoring system isn't appropriate for children. It lists factors in your medical history that promote the growth of *Candida albicans* (Section A), and symptoms commonly found in individuals with yeast-connected illness (Sections B and C).

For each "Yes" answer in Section A, circle the point score in the box at the end of the section. Then move on to Sections B and C and score as directed.

Filling out and scoring the questionnaire should help you and your doctor evaluate the possible role of candida in contributing to your health problems. Yet it will not provide an automatic "Yes" or "No" answer.

SECTION A: HISTORY   POINT SCORE: _____

(1) Have you taken tetracyclines (Sumycin, Panmycin, Vibramycin, Minocin, etc.) or other antibiotics for acne for one month or longer?   25

(2) Have you, at any time in your life, taken other "broad-spectrum" antibiotics* for respiratory, urinary, or other infections for 2 months or longer, or in shorter courses 4 or more times in a 1-year period?   20

(3) Have you taken a broad-spectrum antibiotic*—even in a single course?   6

(4) Have you, at any time in your life, been bothered by persistent prostatitis, vaginitis, or other problems affecting your reproductive organs?   25

(5) Have you been pregnant
  2 or more times?   5
  1 time?   3

(6) Have you taken birth control pills
  For more than 2 years?   15
  For 6 months to 2 years?   8

(7) Have you taken prednisone, Decadron, or other cortisone-type drugs, by injection or inhalation
  For more than 2 weeks?   15
  For 2 weeks or less?   6

(8) Does exposure to perfumes, insecticides, fabric shop odors and other chemicals provoke

    Moderate to severe symptoms?   20

    Mild symptoms?   5

(9) Are your symptoms worse on damp, muggy days or in moldy places?   20

(10) Have you had athlete's foot, ringworm, jock itch, or other chronic fungus infections of the skin or nails? Have such infections been

    Severe or persistent?   20

    Mild to moderate?   10

(11) Do you crave sugar?   10

(12) Do you crave breads?   10

(13) Do you crave alcoholic beverages?   10

(14) Does tobacco smoke really bother you?   10

TOTAL SCORE, SECTION A: _____

*Including Keflex, ampicillin, amoxicillin, Ceclor, Bactrim, and Septra. Such antibiotics kill off "good germs" while they are killing off those that cause infection.

SECTION B: HISTORY   POINT SCORE: _____

For each of your symptoms, enter the appropriate figure in the point score column:

    Not at all   0 points

    Occasional or mild   3 points

    Frequent and/or moderately severe   6 points

    Severe and/or disabling   9 points

Add total score and record it in the box at the end of this section.

POINT SCORE: _____

(1) Fatigue or lethargy   _____

(2) Feeling of being "drained"   _____

(3) Poor memory or concentration   _____

(4) Feeling "spacey" or "unreal"   _____

(5) Depression   _____

(6) Numbness, burning, or tingling _____

(7) Muscle aches _____

(8) Muscle weakness or paralysis _____

(9) Pain and/or swelling in joints _____

(10) Abdominal pain _____

(11) Constipation _____

(12) Diarrhea _____

(13) Bloating _____

(14) Troublesome vaginal discharge _____

(15) Persistent vaginal burning or itching _____

(16) Prostatitis _____

(17) Impotence _____

(18) Loss of sexual desire _____

(19) Endometriosis or infertility _____

(20) Cramps and/or other menstrual irregularities _____

(21) Premenstrual tension _____

(22) Spots in front of the eyes _____

(23) Erratic vision _____

TOTAL SCORE, SECTION B: _____

SECTION C: OTHER SYMPTOMS

For each of your symptoms, enter the appropriate figure in the point score column:

Not at all	0 points
Occasional or mild	1 point
Frequent and/or moderately severe	2 points
Severe and/or disabling	3 points

Add total score and record it in the box at the end of this section.

POINT SCORE: _____

(1) Drowsiness _____

(2) Irritability or jitteriness _____

(3) Incoordination _____

(4) Inability to concentrate _____

(5) Frequent mood swings _____

(6) Headache _____

(7) Dizziness/loss of balance _____

(8) Pressure above ears, feeling of head swelling and tingling _____

(9) Itching   ____
(10) Other rashes   ____
(11) Heartburn   ____
(12) Indigestion   ____
(13) Belching and intestinal gas   ____
(14) Mucus in stools   ____
(15) Hemorrhoids   ____
(16) Dry mouth   ____
(17) Rash or blisters in mouth   ____
(18) Bad breath   ____
(19) Joint swelling or arthritis   ____
(20) Nasal congestion or discharge   ____
(21) Postnasal drip   ____
(22) Nasal itching   ____
(23) Sore or dry throat   ____
(24) Cough   ____
(25) Pain or tightness in chest   ____
(26) Wheezing or shortness of breath   ____
(27) Urinary urgency or frequency   ____
(28) Burning on urination   ____
(29) Failing vision   ____
(30) Burning or tearing of eyes   ____
(31) Recurrent infections or fluid in ears   ____
(32) Ear pain or deafness   ____

TOTAL SCORE, SECTION C: _____

TOTAL SCORE, SECTION A: _____

TOTAL SCORE, SECTION B: _____

GRAND TOTAL SCORE: _____

The Grand Total Score will help you and your doctor decide if your health problems are yeast-connected. Scores in women will run higher, as seven items in the questionnaire apply exclusively to women, while only two apply exclusively to men.

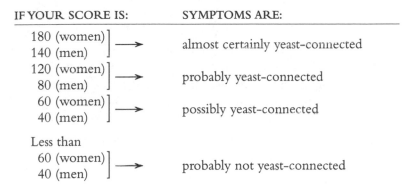

IF YOUR SCORE IS:	SYMPTOMS ARE:
180 (women) / 140 (men) →	almost certainly yeast-connected
120 (women) / 80 (men) →	probably yeast-connected
60 (women) / 40 (men) →	possibly yeast-connected
Less than 60 (women) / 40 (men) →	probably not yeast-connected

Much of the original research on candida was performed by C. Orian Truss, M.D., who wrote *The Missing Diagnosis.* In that book he states that the diagnosis of systemic candidiasis should be suspected in any individual with chronic sinus and upper respiratory conditions and allergies, runny nose, postnasal drip, mucus in the throat, itchy ears, or chronic sore throat. The current laboratory tests that have been most often used to diagnose candida are:

1. The *Comprehensive Digestive Stool Analysis (CDSA)* and *Comprehensive Parasitology* (CP×3—three stool collections over three consecutive days). Rather than simply culture a stool sample for the presence of *Candida albicans,* the CDSA/CP×3 (the CP×3 is the portion of the test that detects candida) is more clinically useful. This battery of integrated diagnostic laboratory tests evaluates digestion, intestinal function, intestinal environment (amount of beneficial and bad bacteria), and absorption by carefully examining the stool. It is a very useful tool in determining the digestive disturbance that is likely to be the underlying factor responsible for candida overgrowth. When the candida can be cultured, the lab can assess which natural and prescrip-

tion antifungal medications are most likely to be effective. In addition, the CDSA may determine that the symptoms are not related to candida overgrowth but rather to conditions such as small intestine bacterial overgrowth, food allergies (sensitivities), and/or the "leaky gut" syndrome. A physician, chiropractor, or naturopathic doctor can order this test for you. (For more information, see Laboratory in the Resource Guide.)

2. *Candida Antibody and Antigen Levels.* Another laboratory method to confirm the presence of candida overgrowth is measuring the level of antibodies to candida or the level of antigens in the blood. The newer candida antibody testing indicates four different responses of the body to candida: (1) whether the person has ever had a candida infection, (2) whether the infection is likely to be currently present, (3) whether the infection has invaded mucous membranes, and (4) how significantly the person is reacting to the antibodies. Usually these tests are not needed, as the results typically only confirm what the patient history, physical examination, and CDSA reveal. Hence, the test does not usually change the course of action. Nonetheless, some patients and physicians may desire confirmation that *Candida albicans* is a responsible factor in the patient's health status. In that situation, these blood tests can be quite helpful and can also be used as a way of monitoring treatment.

Although these laboratory tests are improving, they have not met the current high scientific standards expected for medical diagnosis. This is primarily the reason that the majority of physicians fail to recognize the existence of systemic candidiasis, and many have become antagonistic even to the suggestion of that diagnosis. Unfortunately, this lack of acknowledgment prevents most physicians from ever treating the condition. Although they're not perfect, these tests—especially the CDSA—can still be helpful in the diagnosis of candida. Ultimately, regardless of the test results, a trial candida treatment program has been the best diagnostic test we've had. If there's a definite improvement in your symptoms within four weeks or even sooner, then you probably have candidiasis.

Candida Treatment

Although similar in its holistic scope, the comprehensive treatment program for systemic candidiasis is more challenging than the regimen for asthma or chronic sinusitis without the presence of candida. Treatment depends on the degree of yeast overgrowth and to what extent immune function has been diminished. If yeast symptoms are confined only to the gastrointestinal tract or vagina, the program is shorter and much less involved than if the yeast toxins have spread throughout the body and are causing severe asthma and recurrent sinus infections along with other problems. In the latter case, which is most often the situation with my patients, it can take from six months to one year to cure candidiasis.

The treatment program for systemic candidiasis consists of four components*, and for the best results you should address all phases, I through IV, concurrently:

Phase I: Kill the overgrowth of candida.
Phase II: Eliminate the fuel for the growth of candida through diet.
Phase III: Restore normal bacterial flora in the bowel.
Phase IV: Strengthen the immune system.

*Phases I, II, and III are summarized in Table 1.4, page 21.

Phase I

In my experience, the most effective means of killing candida is through the use of the prescription antifungal drugs Diflucan, Sporanox, and Nizoral. I know of some physicians who have used Lamisil with good results. Although they're all expensive (200 mg of Diflucan can cost as much as $13 per tablet; 200 mg of Nizoral averages about $3) and have potentially harmful side effects, nothing else works as well. They're usually prescribed at 200 mg per day for at least one month. Depending on the response during this first month, I'll either continue daily for another two weeks or reduce to every other day for a second month. Many physicians are reluctant to prescribe these, especially Nizoral, because of possible liver toxicity. Diflucan, Sporanox, and Lamisil are all potentially less harmful to the liver and seem to work a little better than Nizoral. However, during the seven to eight years that I have prescribed it, I have seen only two patients develop the symptoms of hepatitis (inflammation of the liver) from Nizoral, and both resolved quickly after stopping the drug. A blood test for liver enzymes before starting on Nizoral would be helpful in minimizing this risk, as well as taking silymarin (milk-thistle extract), which protects the liver. The recommended dose for this herb is two tablets twice a day. A more probable side effect in using these drugs is die-off, or Herxheimer's reaction, which usually occurs during the first two weeks of treatment and typically lasts for two days to one week. These medications are so powerful in killing yeast that as the organisms die they release a "flood" of toxins into the bloodstream that can cause fatigue, headaches, nausea, loose stools, flu-like aches and pains, and any other symptom that yeast are known to produce. Distilled water, both drunk and used as an enema, vitamin C, and ibuprofen can all help to relieve these die-off symptoms. Although it's possible that for a short time you may feel worse than you did before, you may also choose to look at the "regression" resulting from die-off as a confirmation of your diagnosis of candida, as well as a hopeful sign that you are eliminating yeast and will be feeling much better very soon. Following die-off, most patients experience a level of health significantly greater than they had prior to treating candida. The other prescription drug that's been around far longer than the others I've mentioned is nystatin, available in tablets and powder. It kills candida very well in the bowel, but is not nearly as effective for the rest of the body. When a person has a severe case of candida or grows out candida in their stool and has antibodies in their blood, another option is to take nystatin for 3 to 5 months and add Diflucan, Sporanox, or Nizoral in addition for 4 to 6 weeks. That way the candida can be eradicated in the intestine and genital tracts and then the rest of the body. This is a powerful combination, and I recommend that you be followed closely by your physician. I have seen a few patients require even slightly longer treatments. These prescription drugs are not the whole answer, however. To maximize the benefit of this approach, you must be prepared to adhere to the dietary and supplement recommendations and continue to strengthen your immunity by nurturing yourself physically, mentally, and spiritually.

If you are not able to obtain or cannot take a prescription antifungal drug, there are other available options that work, although they are not quite as effective in quickly reducing candida. Three homeopathic remedies that I'm familiar with are Aqua Flora and Candida-Away (available in health food stores) and Mycocan Combo, available only through health care practitioners. I've used Mycocan with many patients and have seen good results. It's sold, along with a few other similar products, through Mountain States Health Care Products. Thriving Health has another highly effective candida-fighting product. Candida-Free is a blend of essential aromatic oils that are bronchodilating, anti-infective, and decongestive. We've used this product with excellent results in treating asthmatics with candidiasis. It combines essential aromatic oils and herbal extracts that work upon the relationship between the health of the intestinal and respiratory tracts. This connection has been well recognized by traditional Chinese medicine for centuries. The herbs and oils promote healthy gastrointestinal ecology, while their aromatic nature also has a positive impact on the respiratory mucosa.

Another option is to take one of the homeopathics in conjunction with nystatin. There are quite a variety of products available in health food stores that can help to eliminate candida. Most contain caprylic acid, garlic, pau d'arco, plant tannins, grapefruit-seed extract, and other herbs that act directly on candida or indirectly by strengthening the immunity. However, most of these are weak substitutes for prescription drugs or professional products. These OTC anti-yeast products, however, can be helpful following drug therapy and should be taken for a few months after treatment with medication has been completed. This can help to prevent candida from "rebounding." I suggest asking a health care practitioner for a recommendation of which remedy, or combination of remedies, would be the best in your particular case.

A product that I always use in my practice to kill candida is Flora Balance. It is a unique strain of bacteria called *Bacillus laterosporus B.O.D.*, which is available in health food stores or through physicians as Latero-Flora. It has been tested extensively and found to be extremely effective for gastrointestinal dysfunction, food sensitivities, and candidiasis. It is suggested that two capsules be taken twenty minutes before breakfast. I usually continue that dose for about two to three months before reducing it to one daily capsule for several more months.

An herbal combination (made up of more than twenty herbs) that I frequently use as part of my candida elimination program is Intestinalis. It is an excellent remedy for any intestinal infection. While it can be used to treat candida, its greatest therapeutic benefit lies in its treatment or prevention of giardia (a parasite frequently found in untreated water), other internal parasites, and traveler's diarrhea. Several years ago, a woman I was treating for chronic sinusitis and candidiasis went on a group tour to Egypt. Upon her return she was so pleased to report to me that she was the only member of the forty-person group who did not get diarrhea. I'd guess that she was also the only one on the tour taking Intestinalis every day.

The average American diet can cause a thick coat of mucus and impacted food residue to form on the walls of the large intestine. Not only can this encrusted matter affect colon function and contribute to disease by preventing absorption of vital nutrients, it also provides an ideal environment for yeast to thrive. That's why colonic treatments provide another rapid method of removing excess candida from the bowel as well as mitigating die-off effects. Much more effective than an enema, they are best done on a weekly basis in conjunction with taking an antifungal drug. They can cleanse the bowel of candida, toxins, and dead yeast organisms while also helping the inflamed lining of the bowel to begin the healing process. These treatments need to be performed by trained colon hydrotherapists, and in most cities they are not that easy to find. Look for them through the office of a chiropractor or naturopath.

Although not as fast (it can take several months), it is possible to clean the colon by following a candida-control diet, drinking plenty of water, getting regular exercise, and using two natural agents that eliminate colon toxicity—psyllium and bentonite. Mix one heaping teaspoon of psyllium plus two tablespoons of liquid bentonite with 8 to 10 ounces of water or diluted juice twice a day (morning and night). If there is bloating, cut the above dosages in half but still take it two times a day.

3. FOOD—CANDIDA AND HYPOALLERGENIC DIET; VITAMINS, HERBS, AND SUPPLEMENTS

Phase II—Candida Treatment

Eliminating the fuel for candida through diet, while at the same time strengthening your immune system, is the foundation of any treatment program. Even if you're uncertain as to whether or not candida is contributing to your asthma (or your Candida Questionnaire score is not high), I would strongly recommend trying the following diet for at least three months and see if you notice any change in the way you feel. After this initial diet you can then progress to the New Life Eating Plan (NLEP), discussed on page 140. Since each of us has a unique body chemistry, no two candida-control diets will be exactly the same. Also, every physician who treats candidiasis has somewhat different dietary recommendations. But there are some basic principles that apply to almost anyone for a Candida and Hypoallergenic Diet:

1. The diet consists primarily of protein and fresh organic vegetables and a limited amount of complex carbohydrates and fat-containing foods, along with a small amount of fresh fruit.
2. Sugar and concentrated sweets are always to be avoided.
3. Three to six months is a minimum time frame for maintaining the diet, although it can be less restrictive the longer you're on it.
4. It's best to rotate the acceptable foods and not eat a particular food more than once every three or four days. This is especially true of grains.
5. Changing one's diet can be a challenge. The more involved you are in the process—planning, shopping, and cooking—the easier and more rewarding it will be.

The following diet was developed primarily by my coauthor, Todd Nelson. I have also incorporated some suggestions from another naturopathic physician with whom I work closely on treating candida, Sylvia Flesner, and my holistic medical colleague, Ralph Golan, M.D.

Note: The first 21 days, avoid starch and high-sugar foods, including fruit. Also avoid yeast and mold foods.

Foods to Include

Vegetables   Eat freely; 50 to 60 percent of total diet; raw or lightly steamed; organic and clean (wash well); high-water content and low-starch vegetables are best (refer to Tables 4.3 and 4.4, Glycemic Index and Carbohydrate Classifications of Fruits and Vegetables, pages 130–32):

- **Green leafy:** all lettuce, spinach, parsley, cabbage, kale, collard greens, watercress, beet greens, mustard greens, bok choy, sprouts
- **Other low-starch vegetables:** celery, zucchini, summer squash, crookneck squash, green beans, broccoli, cauliflower,

brussels sprouts, radish, bell pepper (green, red, yellow), asparagus, cucumber, tomato, onion, leek, garlic, kohlrabi
- **Moderately low starch:** carrot, beet, rutabaga, turnip, parsnip, eggplant, artichoke, avocado, water chestnuts, peas (green, snow peas), okra.

Protein Emphasis at breakfast and lunch with no less than 60 grams total per day; meats should be antibiotic- and hormone free; fish should be fresh deep-water ocean fish; seeds and nuts should be raw organic. Acceptable proteins include: fish, canned fish in water (salmon and tuna—okay 2–3×/week), turkey, ground turkey, chicken, lamb, wild game, Cornish hens, eggs (limit three to four per week of healthy unchemicalized eggs), seeds and nuts—almonds, cashews, pecans, filberts, pine nuts, Brazil nuts, walnuts, pistachios, sunflower seeds, sesame seeds (ground or in tahini), ground flaxseeds, raw pumpkin seeds.

Complex carbohydrates Starchy vegetables, legumes (introduce after the first 21 days), and whole grains; eat only enough to maintain your energy (try to limit yourself to one serving a day or less); restriction varies according to food allergy, which can be determined with food rotation.

- **Starchy vegetables:** new and red potatoes, sweet potatoes, yams, winter squash (acorn, butternut), pumpkin
- **Legumes:** lentils, split peas, black-eyed peas, beans (kidney, garbanzo, black, navy, pinto, lima, adzuki)
- **Nongluten grains:** brown rice, millet, quinoa, teff, buckwheat, and amaranth; eat sprouted or cooked; organic and clean; available in bulk at health food stores; rotate grains every four days; tasty as breakfast cereals, in salads and soups, in casseroles and stir-frys; store away from light and heat in airtight containers; other whole grains that should be eaten in only limited amounts (they may be allergenic) and only after 21 days without them, include barley, spelt, wild rice, corn, oats, cornmeal, bulgur, and couscous.

Flaxseed oil   1 to 2 tablespoons daily; use on grains or vegetables or as a salad dressing; do *not* heat or cook with; keep refrigerated and away from light; other acceptable oils (cold-pressed)—extra-virgin olive oil, canola, walnut. Use within six weeks of opening.

After 21 Days

Fruits   Introduce fruits into your diet slowly, limiting yourself to one serving per day until you are sure they do not make your symptoms worse. Start with melons, berries—blueberries, raspberries, huckleberries, blackberries, and lemon (only after first 21 days of the diet); then choose from among most other fresh fruits, all of which are generally sweeter than the first group. These include apple, pear, peach, orange, nectarine, apricot, cherry, and pineapple. Citrus and strawberries are strongly suspect as potential allergens with asthma. Fruit juices should be very diluted, at least 1:1 with water. Freshly squeezed is best. Avoid full-strength fruit juices, canned fruit juices, and all dried fruits.

Yeast and mold-containing foods   These are allowable only if you're not allergic. However, I would introduce them very gradually (eat a particular food no more than once every three to four days) and not begin until you have been on the diet for at least three weeks. These foods include: fermented dairy products such as yogurt, kefir, buttermilk, low-fat cottage cheese, and sour cream; fermented foods such as tofu, tempeh, miso, soy sauce. Remember, eating dairy products is generally discouraged for people with respiratory problems.

Foods to Avoid

- Refined sugar and sugar-containing foods: cakes, cookies, candy, doughnuts, pastries, ice cream, pudding, soft drinks, pies, etc.; anything containing sucrose (table sugar), fructose, maltose, lactose, glucose, dextrose, corn sweetener, corn syrup, sorbitol, and manitol; honey; molasses; maple syrup; date sugar; barley malt; rice syrup; NutraSweet; and saccharin; table salt (often contains sugar; use sea salt)

- **To diminish sugar cravings, use chromium picolinate, 200 mcg 2×/day; biotin, 500–1,000 mcg 2×/ day; and a yeast-free B complex, 50 mg 2×/day. Four days without any sugar will also usually eliminate this craving. Try using Stevia, an herb from South America that is a natural sweetener—200–300× sweeter to the taste than sugar, in small amounts. Stevia is non-caloric and does not feed yeast.**
- Milk and dairy products—all cheeses; (unsweetened soy milk is okay and so is butter or ghee, but not in excess)
- Bread and other yeast-raised baked items, including cakes, cookies, and crackers; whole-grain cereals; pastas; tortillas; waffles; bagels and muffins
- Minimize beef and eliminate pork
- Mushrooms—all types
- Rye and wheat (avoid for first three weeks)
- Grapes, plums, bananas, dried fruit, canned fruit, and canned vegetables
- Alcoholic beverages
- Caffeine—both tea and coffee (herbal tea and green tea are okay)
- White or refined flour products, packaged/processed and refined foods; fried foods, fast foods, sausage, and hot dogs
- Vinegar, mustard, ketchup, sauerkraut, olives, and pickles
- Margarine, preservatives (check frozen vegetables)
- Refined and hydrogenated oils
- Leftovers—freeze them for a later date
- Rice milk (high carbohydrate content)

This diet is meant to be a guide. The responses to it will vary greatly, depending on the severity of the candidiasis, food allergies, and the type of medication (if any) you're taking to eliminate candida. The majority of people who closely adhere to it will experience a significant improvement within one month. But suppose you follow it for three to four weeks in addition to

Table 4.3

Glycemic Index

Carbohydrates act like a powerful drug elevating insulin in the body. This in turn can increase fat deposits, LDL cholesterol (the unhealthy kind), and inflammation, while decreasing immunity. The amount of insulin the body produces is based on the amount of carbohydrates that actually enter the bloodstream as the simple sugar glucose. This is why you can consume a large amount of the 3-percent or 6-percent vegetables and fruits (refer to Table 4.4, Carbohydrate Classifications Table, following) in comparison to the amount of grains, starches, breads, or pastas at any given meal.

Example: 1½ cups of broccoli, or any other 3 vegetables = ¼ cup pasta.

This is why it is best to focus on the low-density carbohydrates (3 percent and 6 percent). Not only can you eat more, but there are many other benefits, including high water content, high fiber content, vitamins, minerals, and enzymes.

People are genetically designed to eat primarily fruits and vegetables as their major source of carbohydrates.

All carbohydrates, simple or complex, have to be broken down into simple sugars before being absorbed by the body and entering the bloodstream. The only simple sugar that can actually enter the bloodstream is glucose. The faster glucose enters the bloodstream, the more insulin you make. This is important for you to know when you are making your choice of carbohydrates. *The higher the glycemic index of carbohydrates, the faster it enters the bloodstream as sugar.*

Low Glycemic (Examples: 3-percent and 6-percent fruits and vegetables)
Fructose has to be converted into glucose via the liver, so fruits have a lower glycemic index than grains and starches.

High Glycemic (Examples: bagel, pasta, cooked starches)
Cornflakes are pure glucose linked by chemical bonds. These bonds are easily broken in the stomach and glucose rushes into the bloodstream. Table sugar is one-half glucose and one-half fructose, so it actually enters the bloodstream slower than a bagel.

There are other factors involved that have an effect on how fast the carbohydrates are broken down into simple sugar. Fat and soluble fibers slow the entry of glucose. Soluble fiber is an important distinction. There are two types of fiber, soluble (pectin, apples) and insoluble (cellulose and bran cereal). And because fat slows down the entry of glucose into the bloodstream, the sugar in ice cream actually is absorbed more slowly than that of a bagel. High fiber in low-glycemic foods is the slowest to release sugars.

The more the carbohydrates are cooked, the higher the glycemic index will be. This is because the cell structure is broken down by cooking and processing. The glycemic index is dramatically increased in instant foods like rice and potatoes. Therefore, all bread has a high glycemic index.

Highest Glycemic Index Foods (Examples: puffed cereal and puffed rice cakes)
The body needs a constant intake of carbohydrates for optimal brain function. Too much carbohydrate and the body increases insulin secretion to drive down blood sugar. Too little and the brain will not function efficiently. High-glycemic food should always be avoided with candida overgrowth.

Remember, protein stimulates glucagon, which reduces insulin secretion, while fat and fiber slow down the rate of entry of any carbohydrate.

taking medication and you see no improvement. Then I'd recommend going back to the basic vegetable (low-starch) and protein diet and be suspicious of food allergy. The food you're allergic to is often something you eat every day and have developed a craving for. If you reintroduce new foods very gradually, every three to four days, you should be able to detect the offending food from the symptoms that arise after eating it.

Initially many people complain, "There's nothing to eat on this diet," and it's not unusual to lose eight to ten pounds during the first month. However, there are in fact a multitude of nutritious and tasty choices, and the weight loss will usually subside. A key factor in successfully maintaining the diet lies in finding some recipes that you like. Candida cookbooks are relatively

Table 4.4 *Carbohydrate Classifications of Fruits and Vegetables*
(According to Carbohydrate Content)

VEGETABLES

3%	6%	15%	20+%
asparagus	beans, string	artichoke	beans, dried
bean sprouts	beets	carrot	beans, lima
beet greens	brussels sprouts	oyster plant	corn
broccoli	chives	parsnip	potato, sweet
cabbage	collard greens	peas, green	potato, white
cauliflower	dandelion greens	squash	yam
celery	eggplant		
chard, swiss	kale		
cucumber	kohlrabi		
endive	leek		
lettuce	okra		
mustard greens	onion		
radish	parsley		
spinach	pepper, red		
watercress	pimento		
	pumpkin		
	rutabagas		
	turnip		

FRUITS

3%	6%	15%	20+%
cantaloupe	apricot (fresh only)	apple	banana
melons	blackberries	grapes	figs
rhubarb	blueberries	kumquats	prunes
strawberries	cherries	loganberries	or any dried
tomato	cranberries	mango	fruit
watermelon	grapefruit	mulberries	
	guava	pear	
	kiwi	pineapple (fresh)	
	melons	pomegranate	
	lemon		
	lime		
	orange		
	papaya		
	peach		
	plum		
	raspberries		
	tangerine		

easy to locate in most health food stores. Gail Burton's *Candida Control Cookbook,* Dr. Crook's *The Yeast Connection Cook Book,* Vicki Glassburn's *Who Killed Candida?* and Dr. B. Semon's *Feast Without Yeast* are all excellent resources. The menu and recipe suggestions that follow have been provided by Dr. Todd Nelson.

Menu Suggestions for a Candida Hypoallergenic Diet

★ = recipe included in Appendix
★★ = at health food store

Breakfast Suggestions

- nongluten whole-grain porridge★ (add nuts, seeds, or soy)
- nongluten whole-grain hot cereal★ (add nuts —use stevia for sweetener)
- steamed or lightly sautéed vegetables with poached eggs on top
- fish and steamed vegetables with flaxseed oil
- 12 raw almonds, walnuts, filberts, pecans, or pine nuts
- small handful of raw sunflower seeds or pumpkin seeds
- ground raw sesame or flaxseeds sprinkled on hot cereal
- nut butter or nut milk★
- steamed vegetables
- nut milk smoothie★
- plain soy milk smoothie
- lightly scrambled organic eggs with vegetables
- omelet with vegetables

After 21 days:

Nongluten, nonyeasted pancakes such as amaranth. Add eggs and soy flour, if you are not allergic, for extra protein.
(Also refer to "Nongluten Grains" and Recipes in Appendix.)

Lunch Suggestions

(Protein/vegetable combinations)
- fresh green salad with raw nuts or seeds
- fresh green salad with turkey, fish, lamb, beef, or chicken

- fresh green salad with sprouted beans or cooked beans
- steamed vegetables sprinkled with ground-up raw nuts or seeds
- steamed vegetables and an animal protein
- steamed vegetables or salad and bean, lentil, or pea soup★
- vegetable and nut stir-fry (no rice)
- vegetable and animal protein stir-fry (some rice is allowable)
- fresh tuna salad with mayo or almond mayo from health food store
- vegetable and animal protein soup
- vegetable and bean soup
- vegetable soup or stew★
- fresh vegetable sticks and nut butter for dip
- fresh vegetables and hummus for dip★★
- steamed asparagus wrapped in thinly sliced turkey breast
- turkey or chicken drumsticks and vegetables

Dinner Suggestions
(Complex carbohydrate/vegetable combinations; add nuts and seeds or protein if needed.)
(Refer to nongluten grain recipes)
- vegetable and nongluten whole-grain casserole★
- vegetable and nongluten whole-grain salad★
- vegetable and nongluten whole-grain soup★
- vegetable nori rolls with no mustard★★
- steamed vegetables or green salad with new red potatoes
- vegetables and baked squash or sweet potatoes
- vegetables with beans and rice
- vegetable stir-fry with a nongluten whole grain
★• nongluten pasta salad
★• nongluten pasta with dairy-free pesto sauce★★ and vegetables
- mashed potatoes and vegetables with flax oil and herbs
- stuffed peppers with a nongluten whole-grain and vegetables★
- dairy-free new red potato salad with vegetables

★*Note:* Avoid pasta for the first 21 days.

Beverages
- herb teas, noncitrus
- fresh organic vegetable juice diluted 50 percent★★ (after 2 weeks on the diet)
- pure water
- fresh grated gingerroot tea

Flavorings
- flax oil for salad dressings or in place of butter on steamed vegetables or cooked grains
- cold-pressed olive oil or sesame oil (Omega Nutrition)
- Bragg Liquid Amino Seasoning★★ as a salt substitute (a non-fermented soy sauce)
- fresh lemon, lime, in dressings or on steamed vegetables
- fresh herbs: cilantro, mint, basil, dill, parsley, or rosemary to flavor salads and grains
- fresh spices★★ (avoid table salt and black pepper)
- use ghee instead of margarine or butter
- garlic (great for candida diets)
- gingerroot
- nut butter for sauces and dressings
- sea salt (use sparingly)

Snack Suggestions
- organic vegetable sticks
- raw organic almonds, walnuts, filberts, pine nuts, sunflower seeds, or pumpkin seeds
- nonyeast rye crackers or vegetable sticks with raw nut butter (after 21 days)
- nut milk★
- hummus★★
- nori roll★★
- baked acorn squash
- celery sticks stuffed with mayo-free tuna salad
- cup of bean soup
- nongluten waffle★★ toasted with almond butter (after 21 days)

Phase III

The best way to restore normal bacterial flora in the bowel is through the administration of acidophilus bacteria. This should be done concurrent with Phase I and II (diet) of the treatment program. The friendly intestinal bacteria can be restored through a multitude of *Lactobacillus acidophilus* and *bifidus* products available in health food stores. These can be found in liquids, powders, capsules, and tablets. There are new and better strains being developed on a regular basis, with a wide variety of potency. While there are many brands of acidophilus and bifidus sold in health food stores, most of these actually contain only a small amount of *living* organisms because these products lack the nutrients necessary for survival. Even freeze-dried types usually contain insufficient amounts of acidophilus at the time of use, despite the billions-of-organisms-per-gram content at the time of bottling. To assure potency, follow these guidelines:

1. Buy only refrigerated brands that clearly state an expiration date between one and ten months from the date the item is purchased.
2. Buy either liquid cultures (such as yogurt culture) or powdered forms containing whey (dairy) or nondairy varieties. Lactobacilli are living organisms, and only these forms provide an ample food supply with which to sustain the fragile acidophilus bacteria.

The brand with which I am most familiar is Ethical Nutrients' Maxidophilus with bifidus. This is considered one of the best products available in health food stores. The Metagenics product Ultraflora, available only through health professionals, is also excellent.

Be aware that many yogurt products do not contain a high amount of viable organisms by the time they reach the consumer. This is especially true of highly processed ones and those with many additional ingredients. Those who are sensitive to dairy products, as well as those with asthma and chronic respiratory disease, should not use yogurt as a consistent source of friendly bacteria. Remember to avoid those brands of yogurt that have added sweeteners.

Phase IV

Strengthening the immune system is a vital aspect of treating candidiasis. Phases I, II, and III can all contribute in varying degrees to a stronger immune system. In addition to what has already been presented, the remainder of the physical health recommendations in this chapter—a whole-foods diet (not as restrictive as the candida diet); vitamins, herbs, supplements (see tables on pages 161–63); regular exercise—as well as the guidelines concerning mental, emotional, social, and spiritual health found in Chapters 5 and 6, will all contribute to a powerful immune system.

If you suspect that you have candidiasis, have followed this treatment plan for one to three months, and still experience little or no improvement, there are other options available to you. If you have not already done so, I recommend consulting with your physician about the possibility of taking one of the antifungal prescription drugs. If you've already completed a full course of one of these medications with no improvement, then I'd be most suspicious of food allergy and leaky gut syndrome. This condition can take close to a year to completely resolve, even using some of the new and highly effective dietary supplements formulated to treat this challenging problem. Another way to assess food allergies or sensitivities is a blood antibody test to check for delayed antibody response (IgG-mediated) by the Great Smokies Lab. This test checks for ninety-six different foods and can be ordered and interpreted by a physician, chiropractor, or naturopathic doctor. It is not a perfect test, but it can be a helpful guide in some people. This lab also has testing for the leaky-gut syndrome. (See Resource Guide for Great Smokies Laboratory.) Ultra Clear® Sustain is the product I've used for leaky-gut syndrome, with excellent results. It was formulated and developed by Jeffrey S. Bland, Ph.D., a clinical biochemist and internationally known authority on therapeutic nutrition. It helps to detoxify the body, feed the good bacteria, and assist in healing the "leaky" intestinal lining. It is available through Metagenics (see Resource Guide).

The other possible but less likely coexisting conditions that may be preventing improvement are: intestinal parasites (especially giardia), hypochlorhydria, pancreatic enzyme deficiency (all of which can be assessed by the Comprehensive Digestive Stool Analysis [CDSA] by Great Smokies Laboratory), *Helicobacter pylori,* inhalant mold allergy, hypothyroidism, adrenal exhaustion, chronic viral infections/chronic fatigue syndrome, chemical injury or hypersensitivity, heavy metal poisoning (especially mercury toxicity from silver mercury amalgam dental fillings), and hormone hypersensitivity (particularly to progesterone). Obviously you will need to work with your physician to investigate these possible diagnoses. You may also be getting reinfected with candida from your regular sexual partner. Men, particularly, may transmit candida without being symptomatic themselves, although it is possible for women to be the asymptomatic transmitters.

You will know when you have completely recovered from candidiasis because you'll probably feel better than you have in years, along with a marked improvement or cure of your asthma. You may want to review your initial list of symptoms just to make sure, but most people have no trouble determining that the candida overgrowth is resolved. Don't allow this hard-earned victory over a tenacious foe to be short-lived. Try to maintain a healthy diet (described on the following pages) without reverting back to excess sugar and alcohol. If symptoms get worse as you expand your diet from the candida outline, you can always go back to the basic core Candida Diet program to lessen the toxic load on your body and speed recovery. You can then begin slowly adding foods again. Stay attentive to your symptoms as you add new foods. Remember: *moderation.* Continue to nurture yourself in body, mind, and spirit, and your immune system will afford you excellent health with no concern about the recurrence of candida.

FASTING OR DETOXIFICATION

Periodic supervised **fasting,** also known as **detoxification,** can make a profound difference in treating asthma. There are many clinics throughout Europe that routinely prescribe juice fasting and detoxification, with remarkable results. Fasting enhances the eliminative and cleansing capacity of the lungs, skin, liver, and kidneys. It also rests and restores the digestive system and helps to relax the nervous system and mind. If you're considering fasting as a therapeutic option, it is best to do it under the supervision of a well-trained physician. Dr. Nelson frequently uses the product UltraInflamX Medical Food powder (Metagenics—available only to physicians) along with a cleansing diet.

His basic approach to preventing and treating asthma is *detoxification* and the gut-lung connection via the mucosal response mechanisms. For adults and children over the age of 12, he prefers a three-week course that begins with the candida and hypoallergenic diet that we've just described. It entails a gradual decrease of potentially reactant foods and stabilizes gut dysbiosis and leaky gut, thereby reducing allergy. This approach moves the asthmatic patient toward long-term healthier eating, helps them to feel much better and to reduce medication very quickly, and dramatically increases their energy levels. Along with the diet, he uses UltraInflamX or Ultraclear Plus depending on the individual. They begin with a low dose and work up to 2 scoops 3 times daily. In the second or third week of the program they gradually lower their food intake to the point where they're on UltraInflamX *alone* for three to five days. He then gradually lowers the dose of UltraInflamX as he increases foods of greater density. This enables the patient to determine what, if any, food sensitivities are present. Although this detoxification approach may seem a bit extreme, it is often remarkably successful in a relatively short period of time. It must be done under practitioner supervision.

DIET FOR OPTIMAL HEALTH: NEW LIFE EATING PLAN (NLEP)

There is not one universal diet that ideally suits every individual. Certain lab tests (including blood type), a comprehensive nutritional history, and personal experimentation (trial and error), along with the guidance of a holistic physician, can assist you in determining the diet best suited to your unique requirements. The following guidelines, however, are self-care approaches to establishing a diet for which almost anyone can derive significant health benefits. They were developed by Dr. Todd Nelson during his nearly twenty years of practicing naturopathic medicine and comprise what he calls the New Life Eating Plan (NLEP).

The importance of diet in relationship to health has been emphasized for centuries in both the East and West. While proper diet alone may not be enough to entirely reverse asthma or diseases, most chronic medical conditions can be significantly improved by a diet of nutrient-rich foods and adequate intake of purified water. Unfortunately, our society, with its overreliance on fast foods and snacks, affords great temptation to stray from healthy eating habits. And even when we do resolve to change our diet for the better, many of us wind up confused about what foods to actually eat and how they should be prepared, due in great part to the steady introduction of best-selling books touting the "latest and greatest" cure-all diet. While such books may be well-intentioned, not all of them contain scientifically supported recommendations, and those that do often contradict equally well-researched published information that made the best-seller's list the year before. As a result, a number of polls now indicate that growing numbers of Americans are literally "fed up" with the amount of dietary and nutritional information that is becoming increasingly prevalent in our society.

A good dose of "common sense" can go a long way toward alleviating this confusion. There is a great deal of truth to the old adage "You are what you eat." The foods you consume become the fuel your body uses to carry out its countless functions. Therefore, it makes good sense to eat those foods that are

the best "fuel sources." This means foods that are rich in vitamins, minerals, enzymes, essential fatty and amino acids and
other necessary nutrients, and that are free of preservatives, pesticides, and other substances that deplete the body's energy and
can damage your vital organs. Dr. Nelson's NLEP is the one I
follow and suggest to my patients. Earlier in this chapter we outlined the Candida and Hypoallergenic Diet, which served to
detoxify, while reducing candida and rebalancing body chemistry to help restore optimal function and heal your mucous
membranes and asthma. That diet serves as the basis of healthy
eating for those who are experiencing a yeast overgrowth, aller-

Food Guide Pyramid
A Guide To Daily Food Choices

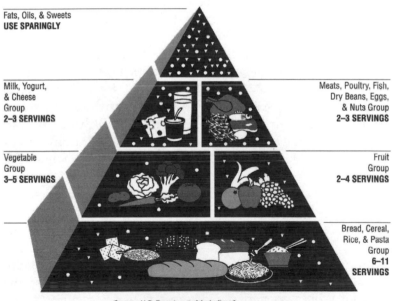

FIGURE 4.9   *Food guide pyramid.*

gies, and asthma. The NLEP, beginning on page 151, allows for some dietary expansion and food rotation.

RETHINKING THE AMERICAN WAY OF EATING

In January 1992, the U.S. Department of Agriculture (USDA) unveiled its recommended dietary pyramid as a guideline for meeting these nutritional needs (see Figure 4.9 on page 141). At the base of this pyramid are whole grains, such as brown rice, bulgur, wheat (breads and pasta), oats, barley, millet, and cereals, with a recommended 6–11 servings from this food group per day. The next section of the pyramid is divided into the categories of fruits and vegetables, with a recommended 2–4 servings of the former and 3–5 servings of the latter. Moving upward, we find a recommended 2–3 servings each of dairy products (milk, yogurt, and cheese), and the meats, poultry, fish, eggs, dry beans, and nut group, with fats, oils, and sweets at the top and used sparingly.

While the USDA food pyramid can be a useful place to start, a number of recent studies now indicate that our daily need for carbohydrates from whole grains may not be as vital as our need for fresh fruits and vegetables. A good deal of this research has been popularized by Dr. Barry Sears, Ph.D., in his book *The Zone Diet.* He and other researchers, like Gerald Reavens, M.D., from Stanford University, author of *Syndrome X,* have found that there are a variety harmful effects resulting from excessive intake of carbohydrates, especially those that have a high *glycemic index* (they break down quickly and release glucose into the blood at a rapid rate). These ill effects include:

• Overstimulation of insulin production, which can lead to excess storage of fat in the body, hypoglycemia, increased inflammation, cardiac risk, and diabetes
• Diminished physical and mental capacity
• Fluctuating energy levels and mood swings

- Predisposition to other chronic diseases, including arthritis, heart disease, and skin disorders

As a result, practitioners of holistic medicine now place more emphasis on the fruits and vegetable groups, recommending more servings of these two food groups over whole grains, breads, pasta, and cereal. Flour-based food—bread, pasta, and bagels—have a very high glycemic index. Whole grains, beans and legumes, and most starchy vegetables except potatoes have a low glycemic index and are emphasized in the NLEP. (Refer to Glycemic Index, Table 4.3, on pages 130–31.)

It is also recommended that milk—other than 1 percent or skim—be eliminated, and that your daily intake of butter, margarine, and cheese be reduced.

Beyond the USDA Food Pyramid

Dr. Nelson developed the NLEP after realizing that all of his chronically ill patients were making at least six critical dietary mistakes. These six were part of a list that he identified as the fifteen most common mistakes in the American diet that undermine health. They are:

1. Excess saturated fat, trans fats, cooked fats, and insufficient essential fatty acids (EFAs)
2. Excess sweets
3. Excess refined carbohydrates and insufficient complex carbohydrates
4. Excess alcohol
5. Excess caffeine
6. Excess salt
7. Excess consumption of overly cooked food
8. Excess processed and devitalized food
9. Excess "high-stress" protein sources and insufficient "low-stress" protein sources
10. Excess consumption of foodborne toxins (preservatives, mold, bacteria, additives, artificial sweeteners, colorings, flavoring, hydrogenated fats, heavy metals)

11. Insufficient high-quality, fresh organic produce—both fruits and vegetables
12. Insufficient pure water
13. Insufficient balanced fiber intake
14. Poor food combinations
15. Stressful eating environment and insufficient chewing

Consistently making poor choices in these fifteen areas over the course of a lifetime will usually result in poor health. This occurs from the cumulative effect of increased chemical toxicity, free-radical damage, nutrient depletion, and dysbiosis, resulting in immune, endocrine, neurologic, rheumatologic, and cardiac dysfunction.

Dr. Nelson has concluded that the goal of any dietary program for preventing and treating a chronic illness should be targeted at correcting these common mistakes and establishing a regenerative way of eating for life. This is the primary purpose of the New Life Eating Plan. As you begin to adopt these principles, you'll soon realize that this diet is an essential component of the daily practice of loving and nurturing yourself.

Let's now explore some of the specific steps you can take in committing to the NLEP or a comparably healthy diet. Out of the fifteen most common mistakes, we will emphasize changing the first six on the list above. These are perhaps the most important mistakes that we commonly make, which we refer to as "The Sickening Six."

THE SICKENING SIX

There are six substances in the American diet that should be substantially eliminated—unhealthy fats, sugar, refined carbohydrates, alcohol, caffeine, and salt. These "substances" can lead to a variety of disease conditions. While it is all right to enjoy these substances in moderation, keeping their intake to a minimum can pay big health dividends. Here are a number of reasons why:

1. Unhealthy Fats

The regular intake of good fats, called essential fatty acids (EFAs), is essential to our health. Unfortunately, most of us are getting too much unhealthy fat in our diets. Primary sources of these harmful fats include red meats, milk and other dairy products, and the hydrogenated trans fats found in margarine, cooking fats, and many brands of peanut butter. These fats are also found in many packaged foods, including most commercial cereals, which also tend to be loaded with sugar.

Unhealthy fats lead to arteriosclerosis and the buildup of plaque on the inner lining of the arteries, where over time they obstruct the flow of blood and the transport of oxygen and nutrients to the body's internal organs. This obstruction, in turn, can lead to heart attacks, angina, stroke, kidney failure, and pre gangrene in the legs.

The excessive intake of unhealthy fats are also associated with certain cancers. Among them are cancer of the breast, colon, rectum, prostate, ovaries, and uterus. This is particularly true of the saturated fats derived from meat products.

The majority of Americans eat an excess of omega-6 fatty acids to the exclusion of omega-3s. Omega-6 fatty acids are essential for health, but we are rarely deficient in them. The one exception could be gamma linoleic acid, which naturally comes from evening primrose and borage oil. This could be a beneficial supplement in some cases. Yet if we eat too many omega-6 fatty acids, especially from safflower, sunflower, and corn oil, peanuts, and land animals, we increase a fat called arachidonic acid, or AA. If AA becomes too elevated in the tissues, it triggers inflammation. Asthma is an inflammatory disease and could be aggravated by too much omega-6 fatty acids. Emphasizing sources of omega-3 fatty acids over the omega-6s is known to counteract this inflammatory response. Good sources of omega-3s are flaxseed oil, fresh ocean fish, fish oil supplements, and most seeds.

Obesity, which is increasing to epidemic proportions in this country, is also directly related to excessive fat (and sugar) intake.

Obesity is a serious disease condition by itself, but if prolonged, it can contribute to many other forms of illness, including adult-onset diabetes.

Becoming aware of your fat intake and minimizing the amount of harmful fats you consume is an important step toward optimal health.

2. Sugar

The use of sugar in your diet can pose many harmful health risks, yet the average American consumes 150 pounds each year. This is the equivalent of over 40 teaspoons of sugar every day. The following are only a few of sugar's health-depleting effects:

- Sugar has been shown to be a risk factor for heart disease, diabetes, hypoglycemia, Syndrome X, *and may be more harmful than fat.*
- Sugar weakens the immune system, increasing susceptibility to infection and allergy, and further exacerbating all other diseases caused by diminished immune function.
- Sugar stimulates excessive insulin production, thereby causing more fat to be stored in the body; lowers HDL cholesterol levels (the healthy cholesterol); increases the production of harmful triglycerides; and increases the risk of arteriosclerosis (hardening of the arteries).
- Sugar contributes to diminished mental capacity and can cause feelings of anxiety, depression, and rage. It has also been implicated in certain cases of attention deficit disorder (ADD).
- High sugar intake is associated with certain cancers, including cancer of the gallbladder and colon. Recently, sugar has also been implicated as a causative factor in cases of breast cancer.
- Excessive sugar in the diet is a primary contributor to candidiasis (intestinal yeast overgrowth), which can lead to a host of health problems, including gastrointestinal disorders, asthma, bronchitis, sinusitis, allergies, and chronic fatigue.

If you still feel a need to satisfy your sweet tooth, substitute modest amounts of stevia, pure honey, or maple syrup to decrease the risk of these adverse effects.

3. Refined Carbohydrates

Refined, or simple, carbohydrates, such as those found in white breads, and pastas made from white flour, are another group of health-threatening agents. When eaten to excess, these types of foods overstimulate insulin production and produce the same excessive fat storage in the body that results from eating too much sugar. This can lead to the onset of diabetes and obesity. The rise in obesity among American children is due in part to a diet heavy in sugars and refined carbohydrates, and lacking in nutritious alternatives, notably fruits and vegetables.

Several recent studies have shown that certain carbohydrates previously promoted as being "whole" sources of starch are very rapidly digested and absorbed. As a result, they elevate blood sugar fully as much as sugar itself, contributing to all of the problems cited above (see "Sugar"). Most carbohydrates have been carefully analyzed and assigned a *glycemic index* rating (for a rating of fruits and vegetables, refer to p. 132). A high glycemic index indicates that a food acts much like sugar in the body, while food sources with a low glycemic index are much slower to be assimilated and therefore offer much better nutritional value. High-gylcemic-index foods include: cornflakes; puffed rice; instant and mashed potatoes; white flour products—bread, pasta, pastry, white rice, and rice milk; maltose; and, of course, sugar itself. Foods with a low glycemic index include whole-grain cereals (oats, brown rice, amaranth, kamut, millet, quinoa, teff); legumes (beans, peas, soybeans); high-water-content vegetables such as celery and green, leafy vegetables; pearled barley; bulgur wheat; sweet potatoes; berries and cherries; yogurt; and fructose.

4. Alcohol

Alcohol is another example of a substance that, when taken in moderation, may enhance health, but when consumed in excess can cause a variety of serious problems. A growing body of research now indicates that one or two beers or a glass of wine per day can be beneficial to health as a way to relieve stress and to improve digestion. In fact, studies have shown that complete abstainers from alcohol have a slightly shorter life expectancy than those who drink in moderate amounts. Unfortunately, for many men especially, alcohol and moderation usually "don't mix."

Although most people drink in order to feel better, evidence indicates that alcohol can significantly contribute to feelings of depression, loneliness, restlessness, and boredom, according to studies conducted by the National Center for Health Statistics. In addition, very moody people are also three times as likely to be heavy drinkers (three or more drinks per day).

Aside from the social stigma surrounding excessive alcohol consumption, too much alcohol can also contribute to obesity; increased blood pressure; diabetes; colon, stomach, breast, mouth, esophagus, laryngeal, and pancreatic cancers; gastrointestinal disorders; impaired liver function; candidiasis; impaired mental functioning; and behavioral and emotional dysfunctions. If you are having difficulty in bringing your alcohol consumption under control, seek the help of a professional counselor.

5. Caffeine

Caffeine is a drug to which more than half of all Americans are addicted. On average, we drink at least two and a half cups of coffee a day, or 425 mg of caffeine. Because caffeine acts as a stimulant, we consume it in order to have more energy. But the quick-fix boost it provides usually lasts only for a few hours, leaving us with greater fatigue and irritability once its effects wear off. Typically, when this happens, we reach for another cup of coffee to keep us going. The result is a roller coaster of ups and downs that, over time, can result in a number of health hazards. Caffeine poses an additional health risk for asthmatics since it is chemically related to theophylline and has a minimal bronchodilating effect. Although a large Italian study found that adults who drank two to three cups of coffee daily had 25 percent less asthma than those who abstained, other studies have shown caffeine to be ineffective in treating an acute asthma attack. People who depend on caffeine for treating acute asthma have found themselves in emergency rooms fighting for their lives far more than those who use medication. There are no studies evaluating the effects of caffeine on childhood asthma symptoms.

While caffeine in moderation (200 mg or less per day) is relatively safe, the regular consumption of greater amounts can result in elevated blood pressure; increased risk of cancer, heart disease, and osteoporosis; poor sleep patterns; anxiety and irritability; dizziness; impaired circulation; urinary frequency, and gastrointestinal disorders. Caffeine also causes loss of calcium from muscle cells and can interfere with the blood-clotting process by decreasing platelet stickiness.

Taken in moderation, however, caffeine has been shown to enhance mental functioning and to improve both alertness and mood, suggesting that 200 mg or less of caffeine per day may be safely tolerated by most individuals.

If you consider yourself addicted to caffeine, the best way to break your habit is to reduce your intake *very gradually,* over a period of a few weeks or even months. Start by substituting noncaffeinated drinks such as herbal tea or a roasted grain beverage in place of one of your normal cups of coffee per day. Over time, cut back further while increasing the number of substitute beverages, and beware of possible withdrawal symptoms such as headache, nervousness, and irritability. Typically, these will pass within a day or two. Also avoid other caffeine sources, such as soft drinks (particularly colas), cocoa, chocolate, and nonherbal teas. If you still choose to drink coffee, the least harmful choice is Swiss water-processed organic decaffeinated coffee.

Table 4.5

Caffeine Amounts (mg)

COFFEE (5-OUNCE CUP)
Decaffeinated instant: 2
Decaffeinated brewed: 2–5
Instant: 65–100
Percolated: 65–125
Drip: 115–175

TEA (5-OUNCE CUP)
Bag, brewed for five minutes: 20–60
Bag, brewed for one minute: 10–40
Loose, black, five-minute brew: 20–85
Loose, green, five-minute brew: 15–80
Iced: 25 to 70

SOFT DRINKS (12-OUNCE GLASS)
Cola: 45
Mountain Dew: 55

CHOCOLATE
Cocoa, 5-ounce cup: 4–6
Milk chocolate, 1 ounce: 3–6
Bittersweet chocolate, 1 ounce: 25–35

6. Salt

Salt is another ingredient that is far too prevalent in many diets, and it poses particular dangers for certain people who suffer from high blood pressure. Many of us have been conditioned since childhood to crave salt, but its overuse draws water into the bloodstream. This, in turn, increases blood volume, causing higher blood pressure levels. Too much salt also upsets the body's sodium-potassium balance, thereby interfering with the lymphatic system's ability to draw wastes away from the cells.

Although some salt can be used in cooking, a good rule of thumb is to avoid adding salt to your food once it is served.

BEGINNING THE NLEP

As a starting point in changing your diet, reduce your intake of red meat, and when you do eat it, choose only the leanest cuts. In its place, have two to three servings per day of either, fish, poultry, healthy eggs, beans, or nuts. Also avoid all cooking fats and oils derived from animal products and those from vegetable sources that are hydrogenated and found in most margarines, many brands of peanut butter, and hydrogenated cooking fats. Instead, use vegetable oils, such as olive or canola. Flaxseed oil, a particularly rich source of vital omega-3 essential fatty acids, can also be used for healthy dressings (but not for cooking). The best oils are from whole vegetables and grains that are un-processed, polyunsaturated, and non-oxidized.

Also pay attention to the various food additives that are commonly found in the typical American diet. These include all chemical preservatives, such as BHA, BHT, sodium nitrate, and sulfites; artificial coloring agents; and artificial sweeteners, such as saccharin, aspartame (NutraSweet), and cyclamates. These additives have the potential to be enormous health risks. To avoid their use, stay away from processed or canned foods and get in the habit of reading labels whenever you go shopping. As a rule, if you can't pronounce the ingredient, don't eat it.

Finally, if you aren't already in the habit of doing so, consider selecting fruits and vegetables that are grown organically, and meats and poultry derived from animals that are raised free-range and are chemical-free. In the former case, you will be eat-ing foods that are richer in nutrients and free of pesticides, artificial fertilizers, preservatives, and other additives. Free-range meats and poultry are the end products of animals that are not subject to injections of growth hormones, antibiotics, and irra-diation commonly found in meats and poultry raised commer-cially.

What follows, by category, are listings of a variety of nutri-tious foods that can be added to your diet for their rich nutrient value.

Vital Abundance, by Karen Falbo, is an excellent cookbook

filled with tasty, healthy recipes that come very close to complying with the NLEP principles. (Refer to the Appendix for some of these recipes.)

FRUITS AND VEGETABLES

Fresh fruits and vegetables, organic when possible, should be a staple of your daily diet as a primary source of carbohydrates. Not only are they rich with nutrients, they also possess vital cleansing properties and high fiber content, which help rid the body of waste and toxins, creating greater levels of energy. Be sure to eat at least part of your daily servings of fruits and vegetables raw, since in this form you will be receiving the highest nutrient content. Lightly steaming vegetables is another healthy way to prepare them. Boiling or overcooking vegetables, on the other hand, can destroy the abundant vitamins, minerals, and enzymes in these foods. Have a goal of eating three to six cups of vegetables daily, mostly at lunch and dinner. In addition eat two to three servings of fruit between meals as snacks.

Among the fruits and vegetables with the greatest nutritional value (especially vitamin C and carotenes) are: blueberries, cherries, red grapes, plums, oranges, cantaloupe, strawberries, apples, guavas, red chili peppers, red and green sweet peppers, kale, parsley, greens (mustard, collard, and turnip), broccoli, cauliflower, brussels sprouts, carrots, yams, spinach, mangoes, winter squash, romaine lettuce, asparagus, tomatoes, onions, garlic, mushrooms, peaches, papayas, bananas, watermelon, and sprouts. *Note: Although they are extremely rich sources of vitamins, minerals, and fiber, fruits impede the digestion of other foods and are therefore best eaten away from meals as snacks: 10 or more minutes before or 2 hours after a meal.*

WHOLE GRAINS AND COMPLEX CARBOYDRATES

Whenever possible, whole grains, beans, and legumes should be a primary source of carbohydrates, as they, too, provide many essential vitamins and minerals. Most grains also supply about 10 percent of excellent-quality protein. Among the recommended whole grains are: amaranth, millet, brown rice, basmati rice, quinoa, barley, rye, oats, and the little-known grain teff. Use wheat sparingly on a rotation basis according to NLEP Phase II. Other sources of complex carbodyrates are starchy vegetables and legumes. Complex carbohydrates provide sustained boosts of energy and digest slowly, releasing their sugars into the bloodstream gradually. This gradual release of sugars helps to maintain insulin balance and contributes to the production of *adenosine triphosphate* (ATP) in the cells, thereby strengthening the immune system. Good sources of starchy vegetables include: sweet potatoes, yams, acorn and butternut squash, carrots, and pumpkins. For legumes, choose black beans, garbanzo beans (chickpeas), lima beans, aduki beans, navy beans, kidney beans, lentils, black-eyed peas, or split peas.

PROTEINS

Proteins are the nutrients your body uses to build cells, repair tissue, and produce the basic building blocks of DNA and RNA. Bones, hair, nails, muscle fibers, collagen and other connective tissues are all composed of protein, and protein itself is second only to water in terms of the body's overall composition.

The main sources of protein for a healthy diet are: fish, chicken and turkey (select cuts that are free-range and free of hormones and antibiotics), healthy eggs (especially those with a high DHA fat content from chickens that have been fed a special brown algae), soy products (organic non-genetically modified soy milk, tofu, miso, and tempeh), sunflower seeds, almonds, cashews, peanuts, pine nuts, pecans, walnuts, and sesame seeds.

Red meats and dairy products are not on this list due to their higher concentration of unhealthy fats, which can contribute to inflammation, and to a host of disease conditions, especially heart disease and hardening of the arteries. Low- or nonfat organic cultured dairy products such as yogurt and cottage cheese are well tolerated by many people.

FATS AND OILS

Contrary to popular belief, all of us need a certain amount of fat in our diet. Fats supply energy reserves that the body draws upon when not enough fat is present in the foods we eat. Fats also serve as a primary form of insulation and help to maintain normal body temperature. In addition, fats help to transport oxygen; absorb fat-soluble vitamins (A, D, E and K); nourish the skin, mucous membranes, and nerves; and serve as an anti-inflammatory. Healthy fat is utilized by the body in the form of essential fatty acids (EFAs).

Excessive fat intake, however, can contribute to a variety of illnesses, especially obesity and heart disease. Fat intake that is too low can also pose health risks. One of the keys to optimal health, then, is to make sure that you are getting an adequate supply of fats in your diet, and that they are "good" fats, not fats that are harmful. These good fats, in the form of oils, remain liquid at room temperature.

The best food sources of healthy fats are the whole foods from which the oils are derived. These include foods such as nuts and seeds, soybeans, olives, and avocados. Healthy fats in the form of oils include: olive, flaxseed (do not use for cooking), and sesame. Essential fatty acids are found in two groups, the omega-3s and the omega-6s. Good sources of omega-3 include cold water fish (salmon, sardines, tuna, sole), wild game, flaxseeds and flaxseed oil, canola oil, walnuts, pumpkin seeds, soybeans, fresh sea vegetables, and leafy greens. Good sources of omega-6 include vegetable oils, legumes, all nuts and seeds, and most grains, breast milk, organ meats, lean meats, leafy greens, borage oil, evening primrose oil, gooseberry and black currant oils.

FIBER

Fiber is one of the most overlooked components of a healthy diet, with the average American diet supplying only one-fourth to one-third of the amount necessary for optimal health. High-fiber diets are associated with less coronary heart disease, lower cholesterol and triglyceride levels, lower blood pressure, lower incidence of cancer (especially colon and rectum), better control of diabetes, and lower incidences of diverticulitis, appendicitis, gallbladder disease, ulcerative colitis, and hernias. Lack of fiber is also the major cause of constipation and hemorrhoids.

Fiber includes the nondigestible substances in the foods that we eat. Good sources of fiber include fruits; the bran portion of whole grains, such as whole wheat, rolled oats, and brown rice; raw and cooked green, yellow and starchy vegetables, such as spinach, romaine lettuce, squash, carrots, beans, and lentils. The goal is 25–35 grams of fiber intake per day.

THE NEW LIFE EATING PLAN

Now that you have been on the Candida and Hypoallergenic Diet for at least three months, you are ready to expand your food choices. Hopefully you have been able to stick to this restricted diet very closely and are reaping the benefits of renewed vitality, less difficulty breathing, reduced medication, better digestion, and an enthusiastic commitment to your self-care. At this point it is natural for you to desire more variety in your food choices. But be careful! Many people will experience great results from eating like this and then adopt the attitude, "I've been doing well, so now I can go back to some of the old foods that I love." In fact, you might be tempted to go overboard in the opposite direction. The worst that can happen is that you will start wheezing again. This is simply your body wisely reminding you to get back to a healthy diet. Let's now look at a safe, gradual way to expand your choices, while continuing to minimize toxicity and allergic reactions, and maximize nutrient density.

At this point in your Asthma Survival Program try allowing the following list of foods back into your diet. Allow them only one at a time every four to six days so you can be more aware of symptoms and track any food reactions. Score your symptoms each day on the symptom chart. If your symptoms seem to increase within a 24- to 72-hour period, and you haven't made any other significant dietary changes, then you are probably reacting to that new food and should continue to avoid it. If you are unsure, keep that food out of your diet for 7 days and retest it.

Once you know you can tolerate a food, allow it on a rotational basis, which means one time every 3 to 5 days. For example, if you have a wheat product on Monday, wait until Thursday to have it again so your body has a chance to clear any reactions it may have to it. This also helps you to prevent developing a reaction to that specific food.

Foods to Test Rotating Back into Your Diet (These are foods to generally deemphasize in the diet and are not required to be healthy. They should be allowed back in only if you enjoy them and you continue to feel well while eating them.)

- Wheat
- Corn
- Bananas
- Cheese
- Cultured dairy: nonfat yogurt or cottage cheese
- Red meat (avoid pork products long term)
- Citrus fruit
- Whole-grain rye crackers
- Higher-glycemic foods: Flour-based foods such as whole-grain pasta, bread, pancakes, muffins, starchier fruits, and vegetables. (Use *very* sparingly.)
- Small amounts of sweetener: Stevia is best, or honey, maple syrup, or brown rice syrup.

Remember: It's what you do most of the time—day in and day out—with your diet that counts. Maintain a lot of variety, so you won't get bored. Do the best you can. Your lungs will let you know if you need to do better.

FOOD ALLERGY

Food allergy ranks as one of the most common conditions in the United States. Compounding this problem is the fact that millions of Americans are unaware that they are having negative reactions to the foods they eat. Ironically, the foods to which we react are the foods we crave the most. The foods that most commonly cause allergy are cow's milk and all dairy products, wheat and other grains, chocolate, corn, sugar, soy, yeast (both brewer's and baker's), oranges, tomatoes, bell peppers, white potatoes, eggs, fish, shellfish, cocoa, onions, nuts, garlic, peanuts, black pepper, red meat, coffee, black tea, beer, wine, and champagne. Aspirin and artificial food colorings can also cause allergic reactions. But as holistic physicians know, any food can cause an unsuspected allergic reaction.

Doris Rapp, M.D., past president of the American Academy of Environmental Medicine and author of *Allergies and Your Family,* recommends the following method for detecting food allergies. Take your pulse in the morning, on an empty stomach. Count your heartbeat for a full minute. Then eat the food you wish to test. Wait 15 to 30 minutes, then retake your pulse. If your heart rate has increased by 15 to 20 beats per minute, chances are that you are sensitive to the food you ate. You may also want to consider food allergy testing as previously mentioned through Great Smokies Laboratory (see Resource Guide). The symptoms of food allergy are many and usually occur within four days after eating the food in question, further contributing to the fact that food allergies are often overlooked as an underlying cause of poor health. Nearly every organ system of the body can be the target of food reactions, including the lungs (asthma), brain (foggy-headedness), heart (rhythm disturbances), gastrointestinal tract (ulcers, colitis), veins (phlebitis), bladder (frequency, urgency, enuresis), and joints (arthritis). If you suspect you suffer from food allergies, consult a holistic physician or practitioner, or a practitioner of environmental medicine who offers a more comprehensive perspective on allergies and food sensitivities than more conventional allergy specialists do. To find such a physician in your area, contact the American Academy of Environmental Medicine at 316-684-5500.

NUTRITIONAL SUPPLEMENTS— VITAMINS, MINERALS, AND HERBS

"I believe that you can, by taking some simple and inexpensive measures, extend your life and your years of well-being. My most important recommendation is that you take vitamins every day to optimum amounts, to supplement the vitamins you receive in your food."

LINUS PAULING, PH.D., two-time Nobel Prize Laureate,

who lived a full and productive ninety-three years by following his own advice

Following the dietary recommendations outlined in Tables 4.6 through 4.10 is a vital step for improving your asthma and creating optimal health for yourself and your loved ones. Sadly, however, a healthy diet alone, even one that is rich with pure, organically grown foods, is no longer enough to ensure total physical well-being. Due to our unhealthy environment and the stresses of daily life, most of us also need to supplement our diets in some fashion. On a daily basis we are exposed to stress in the form of chemicals, emotions, and infection. Chemical stress may come from polluted air and water, food pesticides, insecticides, heavy metals, and even radioactive wastes. More than ever before, foreign chemicals can be found in our foods and environment. Many of these are commercially synthesized, but quite a few are naturally occurring, as well. In 1989, the Kellogg Report stated that 1,000 newly synthesized compounds are introduced into our environment every year. That's the equivalent of three new chemicals per day. Currently, there are approximately

100,000 of these foreign chemicals, or *xenobiotics,* in the world. They include drugs, pesticides, industrial chemicals, food additives and preservatives, and environmental pollutants. As a result, it's very easy for toxic chemicals to find their way into our bodies via the air we breathe, the foods we eat, and the water we drink. We also ingest these chemicals whenever we use drugs (both medicinal and illicit), alcohol, or tobacco.

Compounding this problem is the fact that the soil in which our foods are grown is greatly depleted of the trace minerals needed to create and maintain health. Many of our foods are shipped, frozen, stored, and warehoused, reaching us weeks or months after being harvested. Degeneration of their nutrient value occurs at each stop. Cooking methods, such as boiling and frying, also contribute to nutrient loss once the food reaches our kitchens and restaurants. Moreover, as you've just learned, the standard American diet has become increasingly devoid of nutrients and overburdened with empty calories and nonfood additives. Therefore, even though the body is marvelously designed to eliminate toxins, in today's environment it needs help in doing so.

The following tables appear in Chapter 1 as the "Quick Fix" for asthma. They also serve as a summary of this chapter. In the section that follows the tables I provide you with additional information about most of the vitamins, minerals, herbs, and supplements and why they are included in the Asthma Survival Program.

Table 4.6

The Physical and Environmental Health Components of the *Asthma Survival Program* for Preventing and Treating *Asthma*

	PREVENTIVE MAINTENANCE	TREATING ASTHMA
* Sleep (p. 199)	7–9 hrs/day; no alarm clock	8–10+ hrs/day
* Breathing exercises (p. 87)	Practice 3×/day for at least 5 to 10 min	
* Negative ions or air cleaner (p. 71)	Continuous operation; use ions especially with air-conditioning.	Continuous operation
** Room humidifier, warm mist (p. 80); and *** central humidifier (p. 81)	Use during dry conditions, especially in winter if heat is on and in summer if air conditioner is on.	Continuous operation
* Saline nasal spray (SS spray) (p. 98)	Use daily, several times/day, especially with dirty and/or dry air.	
* Steam Inhaler (p. 97)	Use as needed with dirty and/or dry air.	Use daily, 2–4×/day; (add SS eucalyptus oil)
* Water, bottled or filtered (p. 91)	Drink ½ oz./lb. body weight; with exercise ⅔ oz./lb.	
* Diet (p. 140) * Candida Diet (p. 125)	NLEP—increase fresh fruit, vegetables, whole grains, fiber; cayenne, ginger, onions, and garlic; decrease sugar, dairy, wheat, and alcohol; do food elimination to determine any food allergy.	
* Exercise, preferably aerobic (p. 189)	Minimum 20–30 min, 3–5×/week; avoid outdoors if high pollution and/or pollen, and extremely cold temperatures.	No aerobic; moderate walking OK. Avoid outdoors if high pollution and/or pollen, and cold temperatures.

Table 4.7

Vitamins and Supplements for Preventing and Treating *Asthma*

	Adults		Children (Over 3 Yrs of Age)		Pregnancy	
	(1) PREVENTIVE MAINTENANCE	TREATING ASTHMA	PREVENTION	TREATING ASTHMA	PREVENTION	TREATING ASTHMA
★ Vitamin C (polyascorbate or ester C)	1,000–2,000 mg 3×/day	3,000–5,000 mg 3×/day	100–200 mg 3×/day	500–1,000 mg 3×/day	1,000 mg 2×/day	1,000 mg 4×/day
★ Vitamin E (natural d-alpha mixed tocopherols; avoid if soy-sensitive or use soy-free E)	400 IU 1 or 2×/d	400 IU 2×/d	50 IU 1 or 2×/d	200 IU 2×/d	200 IU 1×/d	200 IU 2×/d
★ Proanthocyanidin (grape-seed extract)	100 mg 1 or 2×/d (on an empty stomach)	200 mg 3×/d (on an empty stomach)	—	100 mg 1×/d	—	100 mg 1×/d
★ Vitamin B_6	50 mg 2×/d	200 mg 2×/d	10 mg 1×/d	25 mg 1×/d	25 mg 1×/d	25 mg 2×/d
★ Vitamin B_{12}	500 mcg 1×/d sublingually (under tongue)	1,000 mcg 1×/d		—	—	500 mcg 1×/d
(★) Multivitamin	1 to 3×/d	1 to 3×/d	Pediatric multivitamin		Prenatal multivitamin with 800 mg folic acid	
★ Magnesium glycinate, arginate, or aspartate	500 mg/d	500 mg/d 2–3×/d	150–250 mg/d	300 mg/d	500 mg/d	500 mg/d
★ Selenium	100–200 mcg/d	200 mcg/d	—	100 mcg/d	25 mcg/d	100 mcg 2×/d
★ (★3) Fish oils (Omega-3 fatty acids)	EPA: 400–600 mg 3×/d DHA: 300–500 mg/d		EPA: 200–300 mg 3×/d DHA: 100–200 mg/d		EPA: 400–600 mg 3×/d DHA: 300–500 mg/d	

	Adults		Children (Over 3 Yrs of Age)		Pregnancy	
	PREVENTIVE MAINTENANCE	TREATING ASTHMA	PREVENTION	TREATING ASTHMA	PREVENTION	TREATING ASTHMA
★ Quercetin	—	1,000 mg 3–6×/day	—	250–500 mg 3×/day	—	—
★ Bromelain	1,000 mg on empty stomach					
† Lobelia (tincture)	—	25 drops in mint tea every 3–4 hrs	—	12 drops in mint tea every 3–4 hrs	—	—
★ ⓧ⁴ Ephedra or *Ma huang*	—	12.5–25 mg 2 or 3×/d	—	5 mg 2×/d	—	—
★ *Ginkgo biloba*	—	40 mg of 24% standardized extract 3×/d	—	20 mg of 24% standardized extract 3×/d	—	—
★ *Coleus forskohlii*	—	25–50 mg of 18% standardized extract of forskolin 2–3×/d	—	12.5–25 mg of 18% standardized extract of forskolin 2–3×/d	—	—
★ N-acetylcystein (NAC)	500 mg/d	500 mg 3×/d	—	200 mg 3×/d	—	500 mg 3×/d
★ Glutathione	—	100 mg 3–4×/day	—	100 mg daily	—	—
★ Garlic 4,000 mcg/pill	1,200 mg/d	1,200–2,000 mg 3×/d	—	1,000 mg 3×/d	—	1,200 mg 3×/d
★ ⓧ⁵ Acidophilus (lactobacillus + bifidus)	½ tsp or 2 caps 2×/d	¼ tsp 2×/d	—	½ tsp or 2 caps 2×/d		
★ Grapefruit(citrus) seed extract (Nutribiotic)	—	100 mg 3×/d or 10 drops in water 3×/d	—	4 drops in water 2×/d	—	100 mg 3×/d or 10 drops in water 3×/d
★ ⓧ⁶ Candida-Free	2 capsules 1 hr after meals 3×/d	—	—	—	—	

	Adults			Children (Over 3 Yrs of Age)		Pregnancy	
	★¹PREVENTIVE MAINTENANCE	TREATING ASTHMA	PREVENTION	TREATING ASTHMA	PREVENTION	TREATING ASTHMA
★★ Beta carotene (food-derived with mixed carotenoids)	25,000 IU 1 or 2×/d	★⑦25,000 IU 3×/d	5,000 IU 1 or 2×/d	10,000 IU 2×/d	25,000 IU 1×/d	25,000 IU 2×/d
★★ Zinc arginate	20–40 mg/d	40–60 mg/d	10 mg/d	10 mg 2×/d	25 mg/d	40 mg/d
★★ Calcium (citrate or hydroxyapatite)	1,000 mg/d; menopause: 1,500 mg/d	1,000 mg/d; menopause: 1,500 mg/d	600–800 mg/d from diet		1,200 mg/d	1,200 mg/d
★★★ Chromium picolinate	200 mcg/d	200 mcg/d	—	—	in prenatal multi-vitamin	
★★★ Pantothenic acid	250 mg/day	500 mg 3×/d	—	50 mg 2–3×/d	—	—
★★★ Hydrochloric acid	10–20 grains after protein meals	—	—	—	—	—
★★★ Folic acid	800 mcg/d	add 1 to 5 mg/d if on oral steroids	—	—	—	—
★★★ ★⑧ Whole adrenal extract	250 mg/d	follow directions on bottle	—	—	—	—

Key to Tables 4.6 and 4.7

★¹Use the higher dosage on days of higher stress, less sleep, and increased air pollution.

★⁷Dosage depends on brand.

★³Use with caution for those with fish allergies and aspirin sensitivity.

★⁴Use only if wheezing is a primary symptom, but do not use with high blood pressure.

★⁵Use dairy free acidophilus and bifidus A.M. and P.M. (empty stomach) for 3 wks at a time, following antibiotics and/or every few months as prevention for candidiasis.

★⁶Use only if candida is suspected and take no longer than 2 months without supervision.

★⁷Use this dosage for a maximum of 1 month.

★⁸Use only if fatigue is a significant symptom or with a history of long-term steroid use.

★ Stage One—begin the program with these.

★★ Stage Two—take these after 3 weeks into the program, or earlier if you choose.

★★★ Stage Three—start these 6 weeks into the program, or sooner if you're comfortable with doing so.

Acute Treatment Options
(only under the supervision of a physician)

In *addition* to those listed in Table 1.2 under the "Treating Asthma" column.

- IV magnesium, alone or in "Meyers Cocktail," during an asthma attack
- IV vitamin C, 10–25 grams, at the onset of a cold (can potentially prevent both the cold and the asthmatic attack)
- IV B$_{12}$: 1,000 mcg weekly, or in accordance with Wright Protocol
- Glutathione, 400 mg/d, either orally or IV. (Recommend Tyler Encapsulations Recancostat for oral administration.)
- UltraInflamX (Metagenics)—an anti-inflammatory medical food powder used for therapeutic detoxification.

Table 4.8

Cold Treatment Program★

- Rest and get more sleep.
- Take vitamin C (in the form of ester C), between 15 and 20,000 mg in the first 24 hours; either 5,000 mg 3 or 4×/day or 2,000 mg every 2 hours, or 1,000 mg every waking hour; very gradually taper this dose over the next 3–5 days.
- Take vitamin A (kills viruses), 150,000 IU daily for 2–3 days; you can take 50,000 IU three times, then gradually taper over the next 2–3 days.
- Take Yin Chiao, a Chinese herb, 5 tablets 4 or 5×/day in the first 48 hours.
- Take garlic, eaten raw (one or two cloves a day) or in liquid or capsule form, 4,000 mcg (of allicin) per day.
- Take echinacea, or EchinOsha Blend® (combination of echinacea with osha root and other herbs), 1 dropperful in water 3–5×/day for 3–5 days; or 900 mg 4×/day. Do not take echinacea if you have an autoimmune disease like lupus, MS, or HIV.
- Take zinc gluconate lozenges, containing at least 13 mg, every 2 hours.
- Gargle with salt water.
- Use a saline nasal spray hourly, preferably the Sinus Survival Spray containing antiviral herbs.
- Take lots of warm or hot liquids; take gingerroot or peppermint tea; you can include ginger, honey, lemon, cayenne, cinnamon, and a teaspoon of brandy.
- Take a hot bath and inhale steam, adding a few drops of eucalyptus, peppermint, and/or tea tree oil.
- Take the homeopathic *Aconitum* (monkshood).
- Eliminate dairy products, bread, concentrated fruit juices, and sugar. Eat lighter foods such as soups, stews, and steamed vegetables; eat less protein.

★ This treatment program is highly effective for diminishing both the duration and intensity of a cold, and works best the more quickly you respond to the first symptoms of a cold. They are usually a sore throat, fatigue, feeling weak or achy, mucus drainage, and possibly some sneezing.

Table 4.9

Candida Treatment Program ⭐¹

- Candida diet—refer to Chapter 4.
- Antifungal medication (Rx)—Diflucan, Sporanox, or Nizoral.⭐²
- Antifungal homeopathic—Mycocan Combo, Aqua Flora, Candida-Away, and several others—an alternative to antifungal Rx.
- Latero-Flora (found in health food stores as Flora Balance)—2 capsules 20 min before breakfast.⭐³
- Acidophilus (*Lactobacillus acidophilus* and *bifidus,* Ethical Nutrients brand is best)—½ teaspoon or 2 caps 3×/day for adults and during pregnancy; ¼ teaspoon 3×/day for children over 3.⭐⁴
- Candida-Free—2 capsules 1 hour after meals. Do this following antifungal medication.⭐⁵
- Garlic, eaten raw (one or two cloves a day) or in liquid, tablet, or capsule form, 4,000 mcg (of allicin) per day. (Metagenics Super Garlic 6000, Ethical Nutrients, or Thriving Health Products)
- Colon hydrotherapy (colonic) treatments.⭐⁶

Key to Candida Treatment Program

⭐¹ To determine if you are a candidate for candida treatment, first take the Candida Questionnaire and Score Sheet in Chapter 4. If your total score is in the "Probably Yeast-Connected" range or higher (above 120 for women and 80 for men), then consider committing to the candida treatment if there is no improvement after 6 weeks on the Asthma Survival Program outlined in the preceding tables.

⭐² Antifungal medication needs to be prescribed and monitored by a physician. If you are unable to find a physician willing to prescribe this, you can either find a holistic physician or consider taking an antifungal homeopathic, although they are not quite as effective as the medication. The higher your Candida Score, the more important it is to include an Rx or homeopathic (or both—the homeopathic can complement the Rx) in your treatment program. Expect some "die-off" effect with possible worsening of your symptoms within the first 2 weeks after beginning this medication, and with the homeopathic too. Recommended dosage for either of these three medications is 200 mg daily for 4 to 6 weeks, then every other day for 3 to 4 weeks.

⭐³ A beneficial bacteria that is effective in killing candida. Usual dosage is 2 capsules daily 20 min before breakfast for 2 or 3 months, then 1 capsule for an additional 2–3 months.

⭐⁴ Begin taking acidophilus at the outset of candida treatment. While restoring normal bacterial flora, it can also assist in detoxification, reducing toxic uptake during die-off, and shorten the duration of treatment.

⭐⁵ Available through Thriving Health Products.

⭐⁶ Not absolutely necessary, but can speed your progress especially during the first month of treatment. To find a colon hydrotherapist, call the office of a holistic (M.D. or D.O.) or naturopathic (N.D.) physician, or a chiropractor.

Table 4.10

Natural Quick-Fix Symptom Treatment

Cough
Gargle, then drink lemon juice and honey (1:1) with a tablespoon of
  vodka (not with Candida) or a pinch of cayenne pepper.
Ginger tea
Wild cherry bark syrup
Bronchial drops (a homeopathic)
Sinus Survival Cough Syrup (with elderberry)
Licorice teas
Bronchoril Expectorant: 2 pills before meals for dry cough (Phyto
  Pharmika or Enzymatic Therapy brand)

Fatigue
Ginseng
Antioxidants, especially vitamin C
Folic acid
Vitamin B_{12}, 500 mcg 2×/day
Vitamin B_6, 75 to 100 mg/day
Pantothenic acid, 500 mg 1 or 2×/day
Meditation
Breathing exercises
Exercise
Sleep
Pace yourself between activity and rest
Rule out anemia

Headache
Adequate water intake
Negative air ions
Meditation
Breathing exercises
Steam
Eucalyptus oil
Acupressure/reflexology points
Massage
Hydrotherapy—alternate hot and cold shower
Garlic or horseradish (chew it)
Calcium/magnesium
Quercetin, 2 caps 3×/day
Magnesium glycinate, 200 mg 2×/day
Ginkgo biloba, 40 mg 3×/day
Feverfew avena, 20 drops 3×/day; or a standardized extract, 1 pill
  2×/day

Runny Nose
Adequate water intake
Saline spray every 1 to 2 hours
Ephedra (not with high blood pressure)
Freeze-dried Nettles, 1 cap 3×/day
Quercetin, 1,000 mg, 2 tabs 3×/day (on an empty stomach)—take with bromelain
Vitamin C, 6,000 to 10,000 mg/day or higher—take as ascorbate or Ester C

Sneezing
Adequate water intake
Acupressure/reflexology points
Freeze-dried Nettles, 2 caps 2–3×/day
Quercetin, 1,000 mg, 2 tabs 3×/day (on an empty stomach)—take with bromelain

Sore Throat
Gargle with lemon juice and honey (1:1)
Gargle with pinch of cayenne + 1 tsp salt in 8 oz. water.
Licorice-based tea (Long Life, Traditional Medicinals, or Throat Coat)
Lozenges (Zand Eucalyptus, Holistic brand Propolis)
Zinc arginate, 30 mg 3×/day—begin with zinc gluconate lozenges for three days, then switch to arginate
Garlic, 2 caps 3×/day
Herbal throat spray—there are many good brands

Stuffy Nose
Adequate water intake
Hot tea with lemon
Hot chicken soup
Steam
Hydrotherapy (hot water from shower) or hot compresses
Eucalyptus oil
Horseradish
Anger release, especially punching
Acupressure/reflexology points
Massage
Orgasm
Exercise
Garlic
Onions
Cayenne pepper
Breathe Right™—External Nasal Dilator
No ice-cold drinks

No dairy
No gluten (wheat, rye, oats, barley)
Ephedra, 20 to 30 drops 4×/day for 2–3 days (max.)
Rule out allergies.
Papaya enzyme, 1 or 2 tablets 4×/day (dissolved in mouth)—use also
  for ear congestion, sinus congestion, and sinus pain
Sinupret, or Quanterra Sinus Defense (a combination of five herbs)

Wheezing
Breathing exercises
Ephedra, 12.5 to 25 mg or 2 or 3×/day (can increase heart rate and
  anxiety—don't use if you have high blood pressure)
Lobelia, 25 drops in mint tea every ½ to 1 hour (may cause nausea)
Coleus forskohlii, 25–50 mg as 18% standardized extract 3x/day
  (Phyto Pharmica brand). No gluten grains or sulfites
No milk or dairy
Caffeine
Magnesium glycinate, citrate, or aspartate, 250 mg every 3 hours
Vitamin B$_6$, 200 mg 2x/day
Vitamin B$_{12}$, 500 mcg (sublingual) 2x/day
Vitamin C, 3,000 to 5,000 3x/day
Selenium, 200 mcg 1×/day
Onions

FREE RADICALS AND ANTIOXIDANTS

One of the biggest threats to our health are free radicals, highly
toxic molecules that play a causative role in many disease conditions, particularly degenerative disorders such as arthritis, heart
disease, cancer, cataracts, macular degeneration, high blood
pressure, emphysema, cirrhosis of the liver, ulcers, toxemia during pregnancy, and mental disorders. Free radicals, or oxidants,
are very unstable and highly reactive molecules that contain one
or more unpaired electrons. They try to capture electrons off
other molecules to gain stability, a process known as oxidation.
They also increase susceptibility to infection and accelerate the
aging process by damaging the cells.

Since free radicals are the primary agents of most cellular
damage, minimizing their harmful effects is important. Antiox-

idants are substances that significantly delay or inhibit oxidation. They neutralize free radicals by supplying electrons. Fortunately, our bodies manufacture antioxidant enzymes within the cells to neutralize and protect against free radicals. Working in tandem with antioxidant nutrients supplied by our diet, such as vitamin A, carotenes, vitamin C, vitamin E, copper, manganese, selenium, and zinc, these enzymes maintain healthy cell function in a variety of ways. As a result, so long as there is an adequate supply of oxygen, water, antioxidant nutrients, and enzymes in the body, cell damage is kept to a minimum. But when our bodies become deficient in any one of these health-enhancing agents, the cells are overrun by free radicals and the antioxidant defenses become unable to maintain their protective shield. This occurs whenever the body's production of antioxidant enzymes and our intake of antioxidant nutrients fall below what is needed to maintain good health. Poor diet, physical and emotional stress, exposure to pollutants, and lack of sleep all contribute to this decline in enzyme production. Escaping such stressors altogether is practically impossible in today's fast-paced world, but help is available in the form of vitamins and other nutritional antioxidant supplements that can offer substantial help in preventing disease, including asthma, and maintaining proper immune function. Allergic reactions in the lungs lead to an influx of inflammatory cells. These cells create excess free radicals by their energy reactions. This then can increase incidence of asthma. Since asthma is a chronic inflammatory condition, antioxidants are a primary intervention. *The most commonly recommended antioxidant vitamins and minerals for asthma include vitamin C, vitamin B$_6$, vitamin E, magnesium, and selenium.*

The following table contains recommended dosages for the most common antioxidant vitamins and minerals, all of which should be part of anyone's daily regimen for creating and maintaining optimal health. Please note that most of the general recommendations are already included in the Asthma Survival regimen presented in Table 4.7 on page 161. There are a number of multivitamin formulas on the market that contain the ingredients listed below, or you can take them separately. Use the higher dosages whenever you are exposed to higher levels of stress, diminished sleep, increased exposure to pollutants and other sources of toxicity, or when you are not eating as well as you should be. Otherwise take at least the minimum dose every day, preferably with your meals.

In this section most of the products I recommend are available in health food stores and some that are only available through Thriving Health Products. You can refer to the Product Index on page 331 for information on how you can obtain them. Many of the studies supporting the use of the supplements that are mentioned here can be found in the References section at the end of the book.

BASIC RECOMMENDATIONS FOR DAILY NUTRITIONAL SUPPLEMENTS

Vitamin C (as polyascorbate or ester C)—1,000 to 2,000 mg 3× /day

Beta-carotene (with mixed carotenoids)—25,000 IU 1 or 2× /day

Vitamin E (as natural d-alpha mixed tocopherols)—400 IU 1 or 2×/day

Proanthocyanidin (grape seed extract)—100 mg 1 or 2×/day

Multivitamin—1 to 3 capsules or tablets per day (dosage depends on brand)

B-complex vitamins—50 to 100 mg of each B vitamin per day

Selenium—100 to 200 mcg per day

Zinc arginate—20 to 40 mg per day

Calcium citrate or hydroxyapatite—1,000 mg per day or 1,500 mg during menopause

Magnesium glycinate, arginate, or aspartate—500 mg per day

Chromium picolinate—200 mcg per day

Omega-3 fatty acids (fish oils)—EPA: 400 to 600 mg 3×/day and DHA: 300 to 500 mg per day

Evening primrose oil—500 mg 2×/day

Manganese—10 to 15 mg per day

Vitamin C

In 1970 the distinguished chemist and Nobel Prize winner Linus Pauling turned his attention to the benefits of megadoses of vitamin C in the prevention and treatment of colds. The verification of his findings by other researchers has been complicated primarily by the great variability in the dosages and types of vitamin C that have been used. In my experience, vitamin C has been extremely effective in the treatment and prevention of colds, allergies, and sinus infections. In that colds are a common trigger of both sinusitis and asthma, their prevention is good preventive medicine. In addition to its antioxidant properties, vitamin C is essential to the manufacture of collagen, the main supportive protein of skin, tendon, bone, cartilage, and connective tissue; has an anti-inflammatory effect, especially in some autoimmune diseases such as lupus and rheumatoid arthritis; can block allergic reactions and rebuild healthy mucous membranes, making it a natural antihistamine; facilitates the absorption of dietary iron; enhances the immune response and white blood cell activity; and, in conjunction with vitamin E, strengthens arterial walls. In a study conducted by researchers from the USDA and the National Institute on Aging, vitamin C was shown to provide greater protection against cholesterol buildup (by raising HDL—the "good" cholesterol) and to reduce the risk of heart disease.

Vitamin C is a powerful antioxidant and as such can be very helpful in combating the free radicals that damage the lungs. That's why it is an essential component of the Asthma Survival Program. There are many studies supporting its use in both preventing and treating asthma. To highlight a few of those studies:

- Forty-one asthmatics received either 1 gram of vitamin C per day or a placebo for 14 weeks. Compare with individuals taking the placebo, those receiving the vitamin C had 73 percent fewer asthma attacks and those that did occur tended to be less severe than in the placebo group.

- Dietary antioxidants can quench free radicals which can damage lungs. Vitamin C can reduce these free radicals.
- In some children, 500 mg daily of vitamin C has a protective effect against exercise-induced asthma.
- Both treated and untreated asthmatic patients have been shown to have significantly lower levels of vitamin C in the blood and white blood cells.
- Vitamin C has been shown to inhibit bronchiole constriction in both normal and asthmatic patients.

The average daily dose for cold and asthma prevention is 3,000 mg. While treating asthma you can increase this dosage to 3,000 to 5,000 mg 3×/day. If you already have a cold or sinus infection, I recommend as much as 15,000 mg a day. Take this amount in divided dosages, either 5,000 mg three times a day with meals (to avoid stomach upset, it is best to take most vitamins with food) or 2,000 to 3,000 mg every two to three hours, preferably as a polyascorbate or Ester C. These are much more easily absorbed with less stomach irritation, and are more potent than ascorbic acid—the more common form of vitamin C found in fruits, vegetables, and most commercial brands of vitamin C. Most vitamin C tablets last for only six to eight hours because they are water soluble. This high dosage for colds and sinus infections should be maintained for several days, or until your symptoms begin to improve. Taper off very gradually over the next two weeks to get back down to the usual daily dose of 3,000 mg. Dr. Pauling's prescription: At the first sign of a cold, take 1,000 mg or more of vitamin C every hour during the waking hours. Possible side effects of dosages above 3,000 mg are diarrhea, bowel gas, and cramps. But these symptoms are more likely to occur with the pure ascorbic acid form of vitamin C. If you experience these symptoms, cut back on your next dose by 1,000 mg. A less common side effect is the development of kidney stones. This can usually be prevented by drinking the recommended daily amount of water or by taking 75 mg of vitamin B_6 a day.

There is quite a variation in the strength of different brands of vitamin C. For instance, 1,000 mg of ascorbate is better absorbed than 1,000 mg of ascorbic acid. Once ascorbic acid is absorbed into our bloodstreams, it reacts with many minerals, such as sodium, calcium, magnesium, and zinc, to form ascorbates. It is in this form, as ascorbates, that vitamin C enters the trillions of cells in our bodies. Taking vitamin C in ascorbate powder is the most effective way to enhance absorption.

Vitamin C, as an antioxidant, is a free-radical scavenger. Studies have shown that our bodies can use a lot more of it when we are under stress. Use your own discretion in varying your dosage, depending on the degree of stress you think you have experienced that day. If it was a high air-pollution day or if you had a rough time at work, take more than the 3,000 mg. The same recommendation holds true for all of the other vitamins and herbs I mention in the following sections. Vitamin C and all of the other vitamins and herbs are more effective if eaten in the natural form of food rather than taken in pill or powder forms. The foods highest in vitamin C, in roughly descending order, are guavas, oranges, cantaloupe, strawberries, red chili peppers, red sweet peppers, green sweet peppers, kale, parsley, collard greens, turnip greens, mustard greens, broccoli, brussels sprouts, and cauliflower. Their vitamin C content is higher when eaten raw. It is also more nutritious (less calories and more fiber) to eat raw fruit than to drink fruit juice.

Linus Pauling died in 1994 at the age of ninety-three of prostate cancer. He reportedly took 10,000 mg of vitamin C every day.

Vitamin A and Beta-Carotene

Most vitamin A comes from its precursor, beta–carotene, which is converted to the vitamin form in the gastrointestinal tract. Beta-carotene is a substance in carotenoids, which are usually found in yellow, orange, or red foods. Listed in roughly descending order of vitamin A content, these include carrots, sweet potatoes, yams, kale, spinach, mangoes, winter squash,

cantaloupe, apricots, broccoli, romaine lettuce, asparagus, tomatoes, nectarines, peaches, and papayas. Vitamin A itself can be
obtained directly from consumption of cod liver oil, liver, kidney, eggs, and dairy products.

Vitamin A helps to maintain the integrity of mucous membranes, is required for growth and repair of cells, is necessary for
protein metabolism, protects night vision, and protects against
cancer. Beta-carotene has been shown to have an effect as an anticancer nutrient—a discovery made by Japanese researchers
more than twenty-five years ago. It is also a powerful antioxidant
and a potent immunostimulator. In research conducted by
Charles Hennekens, M.D., of Harvard Medical School, beta-
carotene was found to reduce dramatically (by 50 percent)
strokes and heart attacks in people who already have cardiovascular disease. Adequate beta-carotene in the diet should supply
the vitamin A you need, but vitamin A deficiency in the United
States is not uncommon. According to a survey by the U.S. Department of Health, Education, and Welfare, about 60 percent
of women and 50 percent of men have intakes below the standard set for good nutrition. Pure vitamin A can be toxic to the
liver in prolonged dosages greater than 50,000 IU (international
units) a day, but beta-carotene is not. The only side effect of
high doses of beta-carotene is yellowing skin, which is not dangerous and disappears when levels are reduced. For treating
asthma, allergies, or sinusitis it is recommended that you take
beta-carotene at 25,000 IU three times a day for no longer than
one month. After the acute episode has been resolved, this
dosage can be reduced to once or twice a day and continued in-
definitely for prevention of all three respiratory conditions and
as part an optimal health regimen.

Vitamin E

The specific functions of vitamin E are unclear, although it is
recognized as a powerful antioxidant and can help protect against
heart attack and stroke. Some studies have shown vitamin E to
raise levels of the desirable cholesterol, HDL. According to Nabil

Elsayed, Ph.D., a professor of public health at UCLA, "You will definitely improve your chances of resisting smog if you increase your vitamin E intake." He believes that vitamin E can significantly reduce lung damage from ozone. Another study indicates that E helps to prevent asthma. For people with sinusitis, allergies, and asthma, 400 IU of vitamin E daily are recommended and should be taken as natural d-alpha mixed tocopherols. When it is combined with selenium, vitamin E becomes twice as potent. This dosage need not be reduced as the symptoms of infection subside. Foods highest in vitamin E are crude and unrefined soybean oil and wheat germ oil, fresh wheat germ, whole grains, raw nuts (most varieties), and all green, leafy vegetables.

A recent study found that eating foods rich in vitamin E may offer protection from certain allergies and reduce the incidence of asthma. Dr. Andrew Fogarty and colleagues from the University of Nottingham in the United Kingdom found that adults who consumed the most vitamin E had fewer allergy-related antibodies in their blood. High levels of those antibodies are associated with asthma and allergies. Since asthma correlates with higher levels of free radicals, an antioxidant like vitamin E can help to lower the incidence and severity of asthma by reducing the free radicals. The study found that for every extra milligram of vitamin E consumed, the level of antibodies fell by 5 percent. The results were based on data from more than 2,600 adults ages 18 to 70 who answered an extensive questionnaire.

Multivitamins

There are many comparable multivitamins from which to choose. Make sure your choice has all of the B vitamins and is yeast-free. Do NOT take a one-a-day–type multivitamin, since their ingredients are usually not scientifically supported and rarely have a significant dose of the necessary nutrients. The multiple should be designed to be taken 2 to 3 times daily with food to assure constant levels of vitamins and minerals in the bloodstream to be available for cellular repair throughout the day and night. Take an exceptional, hypoallergenic multiple whether you have any of the respiratory conditions or not, in addition to the vitamin supplements A, C, and E.

Grape Seed Extract

Proanthocyanidin, or grape seed extract, is a type of bioflavonoid that may be our most powerful antioxidant. It was discovered more than thirty-five years ago by French professor Jack Masquelier, Ph.D., at the University of Bordeaux. It has undergone extensive testing and is considered to be one of the most investigated nutritional supplements on earth. It is closely related to pycnogenol, but is usually less expensive and research has shown it to be even stronger as an antioxidant. While both are natural plant products in the bioflavonoid "family," pycnogenol is made from the bark of the European coastal pine tree and its more potent counterpart comes from the seeds of grapes.

Proanthocyanidin is fifty times more powerful an antioxidant than vitamin E and twenty times more than vitamin C. The earliest clinical tests verified its use for improving conditions of the arteries and capillaries, in prevention of infections, as an anti-inflammatory (especially for arthritis), and for anti-aging. Most European physicians consider it to be their first choice for hay fever, and it is also widely used for asthma. Like many other bioflavonoids, this substance is helpful in treating allergies because it prevents the release of histamine. One 100-mg capsule daily would be a good addition to a daily preventive antioxidant regimen, although I've recently learned that Dr. Masquelier routinely starts his day with 300 mg of grape seed. For treating allergies or asthma, the dosage of grape seed is 100 to 200 mg three times a day. It is best taken on an empty stomach. Sinus Survival Grape Seed Extract, containing Masquelier's original OPC (proanthocyanidin), is available in many health food stores.

Magnesium

Magnesium is a mineral that has been investigated for its effect on asthma since the 1940s. It is a smooth muscle relaxant and can therefore act as a bronchodilator. Magnesium intake (oral) is strongly correlated with asthma symptoms—the more magnesium, the fewer the symptoms. It has also been effectively used intravenously for treating acute asthma attacks. Most asthmatic patients are tissue depleted of magnesium, which has been documented through RBC (red blood cell) magnesium testing, which is more definitive than a regular serum (blood) test. Almost all of the currently used asthma drugs draw magnesium out of the cells lining the bronchioles, which can contribute to bronchial constriction.

Other studies have shown that magnesium deficiency can also increase the release of histamines into the bloodstream, thereby increasing the potential for allergies. Magnesium, in a glycinate or an aspartate form, should be taken orally 500 mg 2 to 3 times per day for acute asthma and 500 mg daily preventively. Thriving Health Products offers magnesium in its most effectively utilized form, glycinate, called Magnesium Extra.

A recent study revealed that children with moderate to severe asthma treated with high-dose intravenous magnesium sulfate exhibit remarkable improvement in short-term pulmonary function along with a 50 percent reduction in hospitalizations.

Alan Gaby, M.D., and Jonathan Wright, M.D., authors of *The Patient's Book of Natural Healing,* have for many years been treating acute asthma in their offices using IV magnesium in the form of the "Meyers Cocktail"—a combination of high-dose magnesium, calcium, vitamin C, and B vitamins. In most cases the asthma improved markedly or subsided completely within a few minutes, saving the patient a trip to the emergency room. They have also used 1,000 mg of magnesium IV weekly as a maintenance dose.

Dr. Wright also promotes **vitamin B$_{12}$** as a primary therapy for asthma. Ideally it is administered IV. He began using it clinically in the 1980s after reviewing some of the clinical research on B$_{12}$ performed in the 1950s. The theory is that B$_{12}$ accelerates the detoxification of sulfites out of the body. Sulfites are toxic by-products of amino acid metabolism and are often found as a preservative in foods and beverages. Researchers theorize that many asthma patients may have insufficient sulfite oxidase, the enzyme needed to detoxify this substance. It is safe to take 500 to 1,000 mcg daily by mouth

Vitamin B_6

Asthma is also usually associated with low vitamin B_6 levels. This finding may be caused in part by some of the commonly used asthma drugs. Both theophylline and aminophylline have both been shown to reduce blood levels of B_6. To maintain and increase levels of B_6, I recommend taking at least 50 mg 2 times per day for preventive maintenance and 200 twice daily for treating acute asthma. In one double-blind study, 76 children with moderate to severe asthma received 200 mg of B_6 daily or a placebo for five months. The B_6 group had significantly reduced symptoms and fewer attacks, and required less cortisone than the placebo group. Results were seen by the second month of treatment. Other studies have shown that some children with asthma have defects in tryptophan metabolism. Tryptophan can produce an excess of serotonin, which is a known bronchial constrictor. Double-blind studies have shown that a tryptophan-restricted diet or B_6 supplementation can correct this defect.

Essential Fatty Acids

Fish oils are well known to reduce inflammatory responses in all tissues by reducing arachidonic acid release, thus limiting leukotriene synthesis and slowing the inflammatory cascade (see page 145). This presumably reduces inflammation in lung tissue as well. In a one-year double-blind study in 1991, 12 asthmatics were given either fish oil (3 grams per day) or a placebo. Lung function, as measured by FEV-1, improved 23 percent in the fish oil group but was unchanged in the placebo group. This improvement was not observed until the ninth month of treatment. This finding supports the case for longer-term supplementation of fish oils in people with asthma and indicates that it is probably most effective in the late-phase reaction of asthma (in contrast to the acute inflammatory response). This secondary late-phase reaction can begin up to 24 hours following the onset of an asthmatic attack and last for weeks or months.

There are many studies documenting the benefits of omega-3 fatty acids in treating asthma. However, fish oils should be used with caution in those with fish allergies or aspirin sensitivity.

Quercetin

Quercetin is a bioflavonoid that naturally occurs in many foods, plants, and blue-green algae. It has been shown to act as a strong anti-inflammatory and antihistamine (which inhibits the release of histamine from mast cells). It is also a potent antioxidant and inhibits the release of leukotrienes, which can be as much as one thousand times stronger than histamines in stimulating inflammatory responses and bronchial constriction. This property makes quercetin an essential component of the Asthma Survival Program and a powerful therapy for both asthma and allergies. Foods that naturally contain quercetin include: onions, garlic, and many dark-colored fruits and vegetables. Quercetin is not absorbed well and therefore should be taken before or between meals and combined with bromelain, a pineapple-derived enzyme at 1,000 mg to improve absorption. For treating asthma the recommended dosage is 1,000 mg 3 to 6×/day. A high-quality quercetin/bromelain combination is available through Thriving Health Products.

Lobelia

In folklore this herb was referred to as "asthma weed" or "Indian tobacco." It has been used since the late eighteenth century by Europeans, followed by Americans, for respiratory illness. Its active ingredients are an alkaloid called coveline, a respiratory stimulant, and lobeline, which acts as an expectorant. Lobelia is a natural antispasmodic, bronchodilator, and mucolytic—thinning secretions and enhancing expectoration. Dr. Nelson has had great success using this herb with his asthmatic patients, especially as a tincture used in children. It is very safe, but in high doses can act as an emetic (induces vomiting). (He was introduced to lobelia by the late noted American herbalist John Christopher, with whom he studied more than twenty years ago.) During an acute asthmatic attack the recommended dosage for adults is 25 drops in a mint tea (12 drops for children) every 3 to 4 hours. Thriving Health Products offers a pure lobelia tincture.

Ephedra (Ma Huang)

Ephedra, or *Ma huang,* should be used only under medical supervision. The medical use of this herb in China can be traced back over 5,000 years! Ephedrine, the active ingredient, was discovered in 1923. Since its commercial use began in 1927 it has had a long history in treating respiratory illness. However, the use of the whole plant is preferable to just using ephedrine, since there is a lower risk of adverse side effects (cardiovascular, especially increased blood pressure), and the plant contains other ingredients that are naturally anti-inflammatory and anti-allergic. Ephedrine is a powerful bronchodilator and decongestant, reducing swelling in the mucous membranes lining both the bronchioles and nasal passages. The peak bronchodilation effect from ephedra occurs in one hour and can last for up to five hours. The FDA advisory review panel on nonprescription drugs recommends that ephedrine-containing products not be used by those with heart disease, high blood pressure, thyroid disease, diabetes, or prostate enlargement. In naturopathic medicine it has been found to work most successfully when used with herbal expectorants and the nutrients recommended in the Asthma Survival Program. The dosage is 12.5 to 25 mg 2 or 3 times per day for adults with acute asthma and 5 mg 2 times per day for children.

Ginkgo biloba

Ginkgo biloba is one of the world's oldest living tree species, believed to have survived for 200 million years. In China, the ginkgo tree is considered sacred, and in traditional Chinese medicine ginkgo biloba is commonly prescribed for respiratory ailments and to maintain and improve brain function. It is also a powerful antioxidant. Ginkgo has been shown to increase circulation to the brain, and is therefore helpful with dementia, Alzheimer's disease, memory loss, concentration problems, vertigo, tinnitus, and dizziness. It can also be used in cases of peripheral vascular disease, such as Raynaud's syndrome, intermittent claudication (severe pain in the calf muscle brought about by walking), numbness, and tingling. There are very few studies reporting ginkgo's usefulness in treating asthma. One small study demonstrated that the standardized extracts of ginkgo's active ingredients, glycosides and ginkolides, reduced bronchospasm and lung hyperreactivity and suggested that they can also benefit exercise-induced asthma. Other studies have shown ginkgo to be of value for cases of head injury, macular degeneration, and impotence. The usual daily dose for adults is 120 mg of standardized extract of ginkolides and glycosides.

Coleus forskolin

Coleus has been used to treat asthma for centuries in Ayurvedic medicine. Its active ingredient, forskolin, acts similarly to theophylline, increasing chemicals in the body that increase bronchodilation. One double-blind study has compared coleus to the drug fenoterol (a beta agonist used in Europe but not yet approved by the FDA) and found it to be as effective a bronchodilator, but without the side effects of tremor and shakiness. There are also two studies that have demonstrated its bronchodilator effect using 1 to 5 mg of forskolin inhaled from a metered dose nebulizer. Coleus is effective taken orally in a dose of 25 mg of 18 percent standardized extract of forskolin, 2 to 3 times daily. To derive maximum benefit, coleus must be taken for at least three months and should be taken long-term. It is difficult to find this herb in a standardized form commercially. It is available through Thriving Health Products.

N-acetylcysteine (NAC)

NAC is an amino acid and an excellent mucolytic agent that effectively breaks up mucus, allowing it to be more easily cleared from the bronchioles. It also promotes the production of glutathione, a powerful antioxidant. I have been using it to treat asthma and bronchitis for many years at a dosage of 500 mg, 3 times daily, for an acute episode and 500 mg daily for preventive maintenance. There are two studies that have shown significant improvement in treating bronchitis, resulting in less shortness of breath, diminished cough, and greater ease of expectoration. Do *not* take NAC at a high dose (above 2,000 mg daily) for longer than three weeks, since it can deplete both zinc and copper. (Both of these minerals should be supplied by your multivitamin.) Some patients in the studies reported occasional side effects, such as stomach upset and headaches, during the test with higher doses, but not enough to discontinue treatment.

Glutathione

Glutathione is a major detoxification antioxidant in the liver. The use of this supplement has produced dramatic results in treating asthma with a dosage of up to 400 mg daily. In 1999 Larry Lands, M.D., a professor at McGill University School of Medicine in Montreal, published several studies demonstrating the benefits of using glutathione on asthma patients. Another earlier study determined that asthmatic patients typically had reduced platelet glutathione peroxidase activity. With a reduction of tissue glutathione, the body has tremendous difficulty reducing free radicals and toxins. Glutathione intake and production becomes even more important when taking asthma medication because of its potential toxic effects on the liver over a prolonged period of time.

Garlic

Garlic, a member of the lily family, is a perennial plant, cultivated around the world, that has been prescribed throughout history to treat a variety of ailments. The Egyptians have been using it for almost 5,000 years, and the Chinese for at least 3,000 years. Hippocrates and Aristotle cited many therapeutic uses for garlic, including the relief of coughs, toothaches, earaches, dandruff, hypertension, atherosclerosis, diarrhea and dysentery, and vaginitis. It can be effective as an antibacterial, antiviral, antifungal, antihypertensive, and anti-inflammatory agent. Its benefits for asthma lie in its anti-inflammatory and antifungal properties. One study has shown it to be even more effective than the drug nystatin in treating candida. At the National Cancer Institute, garlic has recently shown promise in fighting stomach and colon cancer. Garlic is for the most part nontoxic, although it does cause bad breath. Many brand of processed garlic are available at health-food stores in pill, capsule, and liquid forms. Make sure they are standardized for allicin content of at least 4,000 mcg per dose. Raw garlic is best, up to one clove per day. Thriving Health Products carries a highly potent (6,000 mcg per tablet) form of garlic that is enteric-coated and easy on digestion.

Selenium

Selenium is an antioxidant mineral that supports the immune system and can specifically benefit asthma by breaking down leukotrienes, a powerful trigger of allergic reactions. In one study, a group of asthmatics were given selenium daily for 14 weeks and their asthma improved significantly. A study that appeared in a 1990 issue of the medical journal *Thorax* found reduced blood levels of selenium in a group of asthmatics in New Zealand. The absence of selenium in New Zealand soil appears to be one of the key factors contributing to their extremely high incidence of asthma. An article in the *Journal of the National Cancer Institute* said that men with lower levels of selenium in their blood were most likely to develop cancers of the lung, stomach, and pancreas. Low selenium levels might also be linked to bladder cancer. To treat symptomatic asthma, sinus infections, and allergies, I recommend either selenium citrate, aspartate, or picolinate in a dosage of 200 micrograms (mcg) daily, or selenium in a combination pill with vitamin E. Foods high in selenium are whole-wheat products, fish, whole grains, mushrooms, beans, garlic, and liver. Selenium can be toxic to the body, so don't maintain a daily dosage much greater than 200 mcg for a prolonged period of time.

Zinc

The mineral zinc appears to be critical to the release of vitamin A from the liver, helps to convert beta-carotene to vitamin A, and is vital to the process by which new cells are produced and protein metabolized for repair of body tissues. People with asthma, sinusitis, and allergies should take between 40 and 60 mg of zinc arginate daily when symptomatic, and 20 to 40 mg daily for preventive maintenance. The foods highest in zinc are beef liver and the dark meat of turkey. For men, zinc is the most essential nutrient for maintaining a healthy prostate.

Hydrochloric Acid

Studies beginning in the 1930s have shown that up to 40 percent of asthmatic people are hydrochloric acid deficient. This leads to poor protein digestion and upper gastrointestinal putrefaction that could ultimately lead to excess production of hydrogen and methane gases. This situation adds significant stress to the respiratory system. Take hydrochloric acid only if recommended by your physician, since it can aggravate gastroesophageal reflux (heartburn), which in turn can trigger asthma. The usual dose is 10 or more grains *after* protein meals.

Pantothenic Acid

It is well documented that pantothenic acid is effective for improving adrenal cortical function and increased resistance to allergy. Take 250 mg daily for maintenance and 500 mg three times per day while treating asthma, or during your allergy season, and/or during periods of high stress.

Adrenal Extract

Stress, or the experience of asthma itself, and corticosteroids (prednisone) all take a profound toll on adrenal function. Over time, these influences can exhaust adrenal function and generally lower resistance and adaptation to stress. This often becomes a vicious cycle that can severely impede restoration of function. When glucocorticoids (adrenal hormones) become depleted as a result of stress and medications, that result can be general fatigue, hypoglycemia, and loss of potassium. This can then contribute to increased incidence of bronchospasm, infection, inflammation, and slow recovery. Adrenal atrophy is also possible with prolonged stress and long-term steroid therapy. Adrenal extracts, especially when combined with vitamin C and pantothenic acid, can contribute to restoring normal adrenal function. Whole adrenal extract has been used therapeutically since 1931. According to Michael Murray, N.D., they "are typically used as a 'natural' cortisone in cases of allergy and inflammation" (including asthma). The benefits of using adrenal extract are primarily anecdotal, without any good studies to my knowledge. It is important to start with half the dose recommended on the label and build up according to tolerance. The Asthma Survival guidelines are relatively safe. Quality control is essential for adrenal extracts, since they typically are produced from a bovine source. I would recommend Ethical Nutrients or Enzymatic Therapy brand. Do *not* use adrenal extract in children without supervision, and do not use during pregnancy. (The dose will vary depending upon the product. We recommend that you take the dose suggested on the label.)

Licorice Root

Licorice root in the form of tea or supplements can be an effective method for helping restore adrenal function, as well as acting as an anti-inflammatory and anti-allergic substance. It has a cortisol-sparing effect (it inhibits the metabolism of cortisol), but it can also lower potassium and elevate blood pressure if improperly used. However, the D.G.L. form of licorice does not do this. To activate the beneficial properties of licorice, you need to salivate it well before swallowing. The D.G.L. form is available in both wafer and powder form. Take it as directed on the label. Metagenics makes a professional level licorice-based adrenal support formula that is combined with an herb from India called ashwaganda. This is a strong combination and should be taken only under supervision. Stress reduction, sleep, slowing your pace, conflict resolution, and long vacations are also effective methods for strengthening the adrenals.

Folic Acid

It is well known that steroids deplete folic acid. Folic acid is critical in proper nervous system function and blood cell formation. It is also now known to be a protector of the cardiovascular system. If you are on steroids, supplementation is advised. The recommended dosage is 800 mcg daily for maintenance and 5 mg daily during and after oral corticosteroid use for up to two months, under supervision.

Khellin

Cromolyn, which is a mast-cell-stabilizing drug that acts as a bronchodilator, was originally derived from this plant. Khellin is to be used only under supervision and is recommended for treating acute asthmatic attacks. It has been studied and found to be effective when administered intramuscularly. It can also be taken orally in a dosage between 50 and 400 mg. An average intramuscular dose is 200–400 mg and is usually well tolerated.

Under 150 mg is often ineffective. Nausea is the most common side effect. This treatment is rarely being used due to the difficulty of obtaining this herbal extract.

PROFESSIONAL CARE THERAPIES

Asthma Survival is a book and a holistic treatment program with a self-care orientation. However, in treating asthma there are certainly instances in which therapies administered by a physician, conventional or holistic, are needed. It is also perfectly acceptable and not uncommon for an individual with asthma to choose to enhance the results of the Asthma Survival Program with a complementary therapy administered by a physician or health care practitioner. It is neither within the scope of this book nor within our clinical experience to present each of the various complementary professional care therapies that are effective in treating asthma. However, all of the following therapies, administered by a skilled practitioner, can potentially benefit the individual suffering with asthma and can be used as an adjunct to the Asthma Survival Program.

- Traditional Chinese medicine—especially the combination of acupuncture and Chinese herbs; it's particularly effective for mild asthma.
- Osteopathic manipulative therapy—craniosacral therapy is particularly helpful, as are the osteopathic techniques for freeing restricted movement in the chest and diaphragm.
- Ayurvedic (traditional Indian) medicine—includes dietary recommendations and Indian herbs.
- NAET (Nambudripad Allergy Elimination Technique)—an innovative technique combining chiropractic, acupuncture, and kinesiology; well described in the book *Winning the War Against Asthma & Allergies* by Ellen W. Cutler, D.C.
- Homeopathic medicine—especially if practiced by a classical homeopath.

- Massage therapy—one study showed significant improvement in pulmonary function test in children who received regular massages from their parents.
- Energy medicine—especially those modalities that involve touch: healing touch, Therapeutic Touch, Reiki, Shiatsu, jin shin jyutsu, and reflexology; Qi gong can also be helpful for asthma.

4. EXERCISE AND REST

No discussion of physical health would be complete without including the subject of exercise and physical activity. I recognize that for many of you exercise can trigger wheezing, but I also know that if you're willing to make the effort you can learn to reap the benefits of exercise without aggravating your asthma. Remember to start slowly, but be persistent. Research shows that the more asthmatics exercise, the more exercise they can tolerate. Dr. Nelson has worked with two asthmatic patients who became exercise instructors. Regular exercise has the potential to contribute more to the condition of optimal health than any other health practice. Yet, in spite of exercise's many proven benefits, we are becoming an increasingly sedentary nation. This is especially true of our children, who are becoming fatter (25 percent are overweight), weaker, and slower than ever before.

Numerous studies show that sedentary people, on average, don't live as long or enjoy as good health as those who get regular aerobic exercise in the form of brisk walking, running, swimming, cycling, rebounding (jumping on an mini-trampoline), or similar workouts. In fact, some researchers now believe that lack of exercise may be a more significant risk factor for decreased life expectancy than the *combined* risks of cigarette smoking, high cholesterol, being overweight, and high blood pressure. Simply put, *being unfit means being unhealthy.*

The benefits of regular exercise and physical activity include lessening of tension and *decreased* "fight or flight" response, depression, anxiety, smoking, drug use, and incidence of heart disease and cancer; *increased* self-esteem, positive attitudes, joy, spontaneity, mental acuity, mental function, aerobic capacity, and enhanced energy; *increased* muscular strength and flexibility; and *improved* quality of sleep. Regular exercise also results in an increased muscle-to-fat ratio and increased longevity (people who are least fit have a mortality rate three and a half times that of those who are most fit).

Some of the more pronounced benefits of regular exercise occur with older women. A seven-year study conducted by the University of Minnesota School of Public Health tracked the physical activity levels of over 40,000 women, all of whom were postmenopausal and ranged in age from 55 to 69. The results showed that women who exercised at least four times a week at high intensity had up to a 30-percent lowered risk of early death compared to women in the same age group who were sedentary. But even infrequent exercisers among participants in the study (once per week) experienced reduced mortality rates.

In selecting an exercise program, choose a blend of activities that will increase *aerobic capacity, strength,* and *flexibilty.* A regimen focused solely on the strength conditioning, such as weight lifting, while providing strength, does little to increase aerobic capacity and can even diminish flexibility. Adding a stretching routine and an aerobic workout on alternate days will provide a much more effective exercise practice.

Aerobic Exercise

The word *aerobic* means "with oxygen." Aerobic exercise refers to prolonged exercise that requires extra oxygen to supply energy to the muscles. In general, aerobic activities cause moderate shortness of breath, perspiring, and doubling of the resting pulse rate. A few words of conversation should be possible at the height of activity; otherwise the workout may in fact be too strenuous.

Aerobic exercise is based on maintaining your *target heart rate,* producing greater benefits to the cardiovascular system and providing more oxygen to the body than any other form of exercise. To determine what your target heart rate should be, use the following formula: 220 minus your age, multiplied by 60 to 85 percent. Keep in mind that 60 percent is considered low-intensity aerobic exercise, with 70 percent being moderate and 85 percent being high intensity. For example, a 40-year-old's target heart rate is between 108 and 153 beats per minute. To accurately determine your pulse, use your index and middle finger to feel the pulse on the thumb side of your wrist or at your neck, just below the jaw. Using a watch with a second hand, count the number of beats in 60 seconds, which will give you your heart rate in beats per minute (or count for 15 seconds and multiply by 4).

When you have attained your target heart rate—for the average person that should take about five to ten minutes of exercising, but asthmatics should take at least **15 minutes to warm up** to their aerobic level—try to maintain it for at least 20 minutes. It is also beneficial to cool down by working out at a slower heart rate and with less intensity for an additional five to ten minutes before you end your session.

The most convenient forms of aerobic exercise involving the least amount of wear and tear on the body are brisk walking, hiking, swimming, rebounding (jumping on a mini-trampoline), and cycling. Cross-country skiing, if convenient, can also provide a very good aerobic workout. Jogging can also be effective, but to avoid injury, it is recommended that you stretch thoroughly before and after each run, use good running shoes and orthotics—if indicated—and supplement with vitamin C, calcium, and collagen to strengthen your bones, cartilage, muscles, and tendons. Treadmills, rowing machines, stair climbers, stationary bikes, and cross-country ski machines also offer an opportunity for excellent indoor aerobics, as do low-impact aerobics classes. Racquetball, handball, badminton, singles tennis, and basketball provide good aerobic workouts as well.

The keys to a successful aerobic routine are consistency and comfort. Aerobic conditioning does not have to entail a great deal of time, nor does it have to be painful. Find an activity that you can enjoy and keep it fun. Remember, too, that low to moderate aerobic exercise for 45 minutes is just as beneficial as high intensity for 20 minutes. *Do not begin any aerobic activity in the heat of an emotional crisis, especially intense anger.* Wait at least 15 to 20 minutes to avoid the risk of heart attack or arrhythmias that can be triggered under such circumstances. In addition, make sure your aerobic exercise precedes meals by at least half an hour, or follows them by at least two and a half hours, in order to avoid indigestion.

Exercise outdoors if you live or work where it is convenient and safe to do so (specifically with regard to automobile traffic and outdoor air quality and temperature). When you exercise, you may increase your intake of air by as much as ten times your level at rest. The combination of fresh air and sunshine provides greater health benefits than indoor exercise. For chronic respiratory disease sufferers and asthma especially, and for those practicing respiratory preventive medicine, air quality is a critical factor in determining where and when to exercise. Ozone, possibly the most harmful air pollutant for asthmatics, is created by the combination of nitrogen oxides, hydrocarbons, and sunlight. A bright, sunny day in the downtown area of most large cities will produce high concentrations of ozone. The EPA considers air unhealthy when ozone levels top 0.125 parts per million. However, in a study conducted by New York University's Morton Lippman, M.D., thirty healthy adults showed decreases in lung capacity during a half hour of exercise at ozone levels below the federal limit.

I suggest scheduling exercise around the rise and fall of pollution levels. In the summer, ozone builds up during the morning, reaches it maximum late in the afternoon, and then ebbs in the evening. In the winter, ozone isn't such a problem, but cold night air can trap a layer of carbon monoxide, nitrogen dioxide, sulfur dioxide, and particulates that can linger into the early morning. A good general practice is to do outdoor exercise in the morning during the summer and in the evening during the winter. However, if ozone levels are generally high, someone with asthma would probably do better exercising indoors.

If you are used to walking, biking, or jogging along main

roads, lung specialists recommend that you stay away from these high-traffic areas during rush hour. Avoid waiting beside stop signs or stoplights, where carbon monoxide builds up. Henry Going, M.D., a UCLA pulmonologist, says, "I've seen guys jogging in place next to cars at stoplights. You might as well smoke a cigarette." On windy days pollution disperses quickly as you move away from the road. On calm days it can extend about sixty feet from either side of the road.

If all of these concerns pose too great an obstacle, if you live in a highly polluted city, or if you experience a wheeze, cough, or tightness in your chest during your workout, it's time to head indoors for aerobic exercise. Mouth breathing during exercise bypassed the nose and sinuses, your body's natural air filter, so try to remember to *breathe through your nose*. Air pollution can more easily aggravate asthma and chronic bronchitis during exercise. Ozone levels in most homes, gyms, and pools are about half that of the outdoors—even less with a good air-conditioning system.

William S. Silvers, M.D., a Denver allergist with whom I collaborated on the first Sinus Survival Study, has found that many patients with respiratory difficulties who exercise regularly, and follow this with a wet steam exposure, experience improved breathing and increased mucus flow and expectoration, and have less nasal and throat congestion. He recommends that following your 20 to 30 minutes of aerobic exercise, and after your heart rate has dropped to its pre-exercise level, you have 5 to 10 minutes of exposure to wet steam. This can be done in either a steam room at a health club, in the bathroom of your home, with a Steam Inhaler, or by standing over a boiling pot of water with a towel over your head. You should do nasal/chest breathing, which is best performed by taking a deep, slow inhalation through your nose and then breathing out from your chest. Do this as many days as you can, whether you exercise indoors or outdoors.

Moderate exercise is less strenuous than aerobic but still beneficial. In a research project at the University of Minnesota School of Public Health, moderate exercise was defined as rapid walking, bowling, gardening, yard work, home repairs, dancing, and home exercise, conducted for about an hour daily. A tread-mill test determined that those who got this much leisure-time exercise had healthier hearts than those who got less or none. There was no added benefit in doing more than an hour's worth of physical activity. Robert E. Thayer, Ph.D., a professor of psy-chology at California State University, Long Beach, has found that brisk walks only ten minutes long can increase people's feel-ings of energy (sometimes for several hours), reduce tension, and make personal problems appear less serious. Not only does it nourish mind and body, *walking is also by far the easiest, safest, and least expensive (you need only comfortable shoes) form of exercise.* Briskly walking two miles at 3.5 to 4 miles per hour (or 15- to 17-minute miles) burns nearly as many calories as running at a moderate pace, and confers similar fitness benefits. By swinging your arms, you'll burn 5 to 10 percent more calories and get an upper-body workout as well.

Strength Conditioning

Building and maintaining muscle strength is another essential component of your overall exercise program. Strength condi-tioning falls under the following three categories: *Strengthening without aids* includes calisthenics such as sit-ups, push-ups, jump-ing jacks, and swimming. *Strengthening with aids* includes chin-ups, dips, weight lifting, and training on weight machines. And *strengthening with aerobics* involves various forms of interval train-ing that can be done running, bicycling, jumping rope, circuit training with weight machines, and working out on a heavy bag. The goal of interval training is to work intensively, reach-ing your maximum heart level for a short interval, then lower-ing the level of activity to recover. Repeating this process while maintaining your heart rate in its target zone reduces recovery time, strengthens various muscle groups, and conditions the car-diovascular system.

Weight training is perhaps the most popular form of strength-conditioning exercise. To design a weight program to meet your specific needs, consult with a personal trainer, who will most likely advise you to work out two or three times a week. It isn't necessary to lift a lot of weight to build and tone muscle. If muscle tone and definition is your goal, best results will be achieved using less weight and more repetitions. To build mass, increase the amount of weight you use and do fewer repetitions. Remember to breathe *out* (especially important for asthmatics, and be sure NOT to hold your breath during weight training) as you exert effort, and for free-weight exercises it is advisable to work with a spotter. Also, wear a weight belt to help keep your spine properly aligned. If you are unable to work with a personal trainer, refer to the list of recommended books for helpful guidelines in designing your strength-conditioning program.

Increasing Flexibility

The final component of a good exercise program addresses flexibility. This includes stretching exercises, yoga, tai chi, and the Feldenkrais Method. Exercise that promotes flexibility also significantly contributes to strength and function by allowing the body's muscle groups to perform at maximum efficiency. Lack of flexibility can severely inhibit physical performance, increase the potential for injury, and compromise posture. Muscles exist in a state of static tension wherein contrasting sets of muscles exert similar force to create a state of balance. When muscles become weak or inflexible, this balance is disrupted, resulting in reduced function or postural misalignment. Additional benefits of muscle flexibility include improved circulation, enhanced suppleness of connective tissue (tendons and ligaments), decreased risk of injury, and greater body awareness.

Stretching exercises   Some form of stretching is recommended before and after both aerobic and strengthening workouts. Before you begin stretching, do five minutes of movement to warm up your muscles and body core. This will enhance your circulation and make stretching easier. Never stretch to the point of pain. Ideally, you should feel a tension in the affected muscle or muscle group that you are working. As you do, breathe into the stretch to elongate and relax the muscle group as you hold the posture for 20 to 30 seconds. Repeat each stretch at least twice. You should notice that your range increases on the second and third repetition. A few minutes of daily stretching will noticeably improve your well-being over time.

Yoga   *Yoga,* a Sanskrit word meaning "to yoke," refers to a balanced practice of physical exercise, breathing, and meditation to unify body, mind, and spirit, making yoga one of the most effective and ancient forms of holistic self-care. The benefits of this 5,000-year-old system of mind-body training to improve flexibility, strength, and concentration are well documented. The basis of yoga is the *breath,* a variant of abdominal or belly breathing called oujai breathing. This makes yoga especially helpful to the individual with asthma. Several studies have supported this fact. There are a number of yogic systems; *hatha yoga* is most well-known in the West. Hatha yoga postures, or *asanas,* affect specific muscle groups and organs to impart physical strength and flexibility, as well as emotional and mental peace of mind.

There are a variety of hatha yoga forms available. Initially it is a good idea to receive instruction for at least a few months, due to the subtleties involved in yoga practice that are not apparent without firsthand experience of its practice under the guidance of a qualified yoga instructor.

Tai chi   Sometimes referred to as "meditation in motion," tai chi or tai chi chuan, like yoga, is thousands of years old. It involves slow-motion movements integrated with focused belly breathing and visualization and is practiced daily by tens of millions of people in mainland China. The goal of tai chi is to move *qi* ("chee"), or *vital life force energy,* along the various meridians, or energetic pathways, of the body's various organ systems. According to traditional Chinese medicine, when the flow of *qi* is balanced and unobstructed, both blood and lymph flow are enhanced and the body's neurological impulses function at optimal capacity. The result is greater vitality, resistance to disease, better balance, stimulation of the "relaxation response," increased oxygenation of the blood, deeper sleep, and increased body/mind awareness. Although not as well known as yoga in this country, tai chi is rapidly gaining in popularity, and tai chi instructors can be found in most metropolitan areas. After being taught the basic movements of tai chi, you can practice them almost anywhere to instill a centeredness and sense of calm and to alleviate stress. It, too, can be quite helpful for someone with asthma.

Exercise-Induced Asthma

Aerobic exercise was an integral part of the program I used to cure my own chronic sinusitis, and it is still the most enjoyable part of my daily routine. If you are prone to exercise-induced asthma, don't allow it to prevent you from exercising. It would be quite helpful for you to practice the breathing exercises beginning on page 87 on a regular basis. Through trial and error you'll have to determine on your own what level of exercise you can tolerate without triggering a wheeze. There are a number of variables that will affect this level of tolerance: medications used prior to exercise, air quality and temperature, what and when you've eating prior to exercise, emotional stress at time of exercise, and degree of difficulty of exercise. As you keep track of these variables, you become much more aware of the factors that aggravate your asthma. You will then be able to continually modify your exercise regimen to accommodate your own unique condition. This will allow you to make steady progress in increasing the duration and intensity of your exercise. Initially it requires discipline. Start gradually and try not to push yourself too hard. Exercise does not have to hurt to be beneficial, in spite of the prevalent belief in "no pain, no gain." As you begin, I'd recommend using your bronchodilator liberally prior to your exercise. In addition, 2,000 mg of vitamin C taken before exercise has been shown to significantly reduce the incidence of exercise-induced asthma. If your asthma is mild, use a short-acting inhaled beta agonist 15 to 20 minutes before exercising. This will offer about 45 minutes of protection. The longer-acting beta agonist salmeterol (Serevent) is also used for exercise-induced asthma. When inhaled 30 to 60 minutes before exercise, it offers protection for up to 12 hours. Cromolyn or nedocromil (Tilade) inhaled 15 minutes before exercise can offer protection for 2 to 4 hours. Another option is daily use of an inhaled anti–inflammatory drug. Sometimes both types of drugs—a beta agonist and inhaled cromolyn sodium or nedocromil—are used together. If exercise-induced asthma attacks are severe, you may need regular, daily, inhaled corticosteroid medication. You'll need to discuss this with your physician. But whatever your asthma status, it should not prevent you from exercising. Exercise-induced asthma occurs more with allergic people than non-allergic; more often outdoors than indoors; and more often in cold air than warm.

It won't take long before you start looking forward to your exercise session as one of the highlights of your day. The benefits that you will soon realize will help to increase your motivation to continue. You may eventually do it every day, although research has shown no increased cardiovascular benefits beyond five days a week (three times a week is minimum). However, exercise does much more than merely benefit your heart. As these aerobic workouts strengthen your heart and lungs directly, your ability to provide oxygen to every part of your body is enhanced—and this, after all, is the scientific basis of physical health. It will help you to develop the capacity to breathe freely and easily and possibly become the key element in your treatment program to overcome your asthmatic condition. You may also be interested in knowing that nearly 30 percent of the cyclists and swimmers in the 1996 Summer Olympics in Atlanta and 20 percent of all the athletes in the 1984 Summer Olympics were diagnosed asthmatics. Among the well-known athletes with asthma are Amy Van Dyken (winner of six medals in swimming, including four gold, at the 1996 and 2000 Olympics), Jackie Joyner-Kersee (Olympic track gold medalist), Dennis Rodman (former NBA player for the Chicago Bulls), Mary Slaney (Olympic runner), Mary Joe Fernandez (pro tennis player),

Danny Manning (plays basketball for the Phoenix Suns), and Greg Louganis (gold-medal diver).

As a human animal, you can experience many of life's greatest pleasures only through your body. Regular exercise can add immeasurably to your enjoyment of life and heighten your sense of well-being.

Sleep and Relaxation

While diet, the use of supplements, and exercise can all benefit physical health and improve immune function, perhaps the most powerful and overlooked key to overall well-being is sleep. The average person requires between eight and nine hours of uninterrupted sleep, yet in the United States we average between six and eight hours, with an estimated 50 million Americans suffering from insomnia.

Lack of sleep and its resulting depression of the immune system can be a factor in many chronic health conditions and is one of the most common causes of colds and sinus infections. Additional sleep is therefore an essential component in the holistic treatment of such conditions. Besides lowered immune function, sleep deprivation can also cause a decrease in productivity, creativity, and job performance and can affect mood and mental alertness. In cases of insomnia, most incidents of sleep deprivation are due to a specific stress-producing event. While stress-induced insomnia is usually temporary, it may persist well beyond the precipitating event to become a chronic problem. Overstimulation of the nervous system (especially from caffeine, salt, or sugar) or simply the fear that you can't fall asleep are other common causes.

Researchers have identified two types of sleep: *heavy* and *light*. During heavier, or non-rapid-eye-movement (NREM) sleep, your body's self-repair and healing mechanisms are revitalized, enabling your body to repair itself. During lighter, rapid-eye-movement (REM) sleep, you dream more, releasing stress and tension. (For more on dreams, see Chapter 5.)

Conventional medicine commonly prescribes sleeping pills for insomnia and other sleep disorders, but as with almost all medications, there are unpleasant side effects to contend with, as well as the risk of developing dependency. A more holistic approach to ensuring adequate sleep begins with establishing a regular bedtime every night so that you can begin to re-attune yourself to nature's rhythms. By not awakening to an alarm clock, you allow your body to get the amount of sleep that it requires. Try going to sleep earlier if you find you still need an alarm clock.

Dr. Nelson has observed that many insomniacs (those that awaken in the middle of the night and can't fall back to sleep) have developed the habit of "clock watching" during the night when they wake up. They typically have an alarm clock with bright red digits glaring at them in the darkness. He believes that they've actually trained their unconscious mind to *look for* those preprogrammed times. The silent message that they consistently hear (especially before going to bed) is "I wake up every night at————A.M." As this pattern of awakening too early continues, they are literally creating the expectation to awaken at their designated time and their hormones and nervous system follows their explicit instructions. He coaches them on breaking this habit by asking them to never check the time, turn the clock around so that's it's facing away from them, or turn it off! His theory has been confirmed with multiple patients who were able to stop their clock-watching and as a result end their insomnia.

According to Ayurvedic medicine (the traditional medicine of India), the circadian rhythm, caused by the earth rotating on its axis every twenty-four hours, has a counterpart in the human body. Modern science has confirmed that many neurological and endocrine functions follow this circadian rhythm, including the sleep-wakefulness cycle. Ayurveda teaches that the ideal bedtime for the deepest sleep and for being in sync with this natural rhythm is 10 P.M. Unfortunately, most people with insomnia dread bedtime and go to bed later, when sleep tends to be somewhat lighter and more active. Ayurveda also states that eight hours of sleep beginning at 9:30 P.M. is twice as restful as eight hours beginning at 2 A.M. It is also important in resetting your biological clock to get up early and at the same time every day, regardless of when you go to bed. Establishing an early wake-up time (6 or 7 A.M.) is essential for overcoming insomnia. You'll eventually begin to feel sleepier earlier in the evening, and even if you aren't actually sleeping by 10 P.M., you'll benefit just by resting in bed at that hour.

Other natural remedies include:

- vitamin B complex, 50 to 100 mg daily with meals; the best food sources of the B vitamins are liver, whole grains, wheat germ, tuna, walnuts, peanuts, bananas, sunflower seeds, and blackstrap molasses
- niacinamide (vitamin B_3) up to one gram (1,000 mg) at bedtime, for people who have trouble staying asleep, not falling asleep
- calcium and magnesium, 500 to 1,000 mg of each within 45 minutes of bedtime
- chamomile, passionflower, hops, skullcap, and especially valerian herbs; they are natural sedatives that do not alter the quality of sleep the way prescription and over-the-counter drugs do; they can all be taken as a tea, while valerian and passionflower are available in stronger dosages in a tincture form
- kava kava, another useful herb for both anxiety and insomnia; recommended dosage for sleep is two to three capsules (60 to 75 mg per capsule) an hour before bedtime
- tryptophan, three to five grams 45 minutes before retiring, and at least one and a half hours after eating protein; adding B_6 to the tryptophan along with fruit juice can improve results. Tryptophan is available by prescription only.
- 5-hydroxytrytophan (5-HTP), 100 to 250 mg before bed
- melatonin, a hormone produced by the pineal gland in response to darkness, and most effective for difficulty falling asleep; recommended dosage ranges from 1 to 4 mg, one half hour to one hour before bed. Melatonin can also be used for sleep maintenance with a sustained-release 1-mg preparation.

- hot bath or hot tub
- breathing exercises and/or meditation to relax muscles and relieve tension

Most important, don't worry about lost sleep, since in most cases anxiety is what caused the problem in the first place. If you can learn to relax without drugs, you will have cured your sleeping problems while giving your immune system a powerful boost. Nearly all of the recommendations in Chapters 5 and 6 will help you to achieve this goal.

Relaxation is another essential ability that promotes physical health. Derived from the Latin *relaxare,* meaning "to loosen," relaxation is a way to allow the mind to return to a natural state of equilibrium, creating a state of balance between the right and left brain. It is also a highly effective means of stress reduction.

Relaxation is a skill that can be improved upon with practice; therefore, it is recommended that you take time each day to relax. This can be achieved as easily as taking a few deep abdominal breaths or simply shifting your focus away from your problems and concerns, or through any activity that engages your creative and physical faculties. Such activities include reading and writing, gardening, taking a walk, painting, singing, playing music, doing crafts, or any other hobby that you enjoy for its own sake, without the need to be concerned about your performance. Committing two to three evening hours a week to the hobby or activity of your choice will help make relaxation a natural and regular part of your daily experience. The ability to relax and shift gears away from the competitive drive that compels most of us in our society holds the key to greater health.

SUMMARY

In this chapter you have been provided with an array of therapeutic options with which to improve your asthma while you begin the process of experiencing optimal health. You should have enough information to effectively implement the first four components of the *essential 8:*

- Air and Breathing
- Water and Moisture (+ Nasal Hygiene)
- Food and Supplements
- Exercise and Rest

If you are willing to make at least a three-month commitment to this physical/environmental component of the Asthma Survival Program, you will notice a significant improvement in your state of health. I strongly suggest that you work with your physician on gradually tapering off your medication(s) as you progress and deepen your commitment to the program. If your physician is unwilling to participate with you in your healing process, then I would look for a holistic physician or practitioner in your community. You can refer to the Resource Guide in this book and contact either (or both) the American Board of Holistic Medicine (in early 2001 there are nearly 300 board-certified holistic physicians in the United States) or the American Holistic Medical Association.

Your work, however, is not yet complete. This chapter has given you a lot to *do,* with a number of practical steps that will quickly help to reverse your weakening state of health. If you are committed to healing your life along with curing your asthma, you must continue to address each of the factors that have contributed to your respiratory dis-ease. In the next two chapters, "Healing Your Mind" and "Healing Your Spirit," you will learn more about the mental, emotional, spiritual, and social causes of asthma and what you can do to change these aspects of your life. It will usually take a bit longer to see results, but the emphasis is more on how you would like to *be* in this world, rather than on what you do. It is both challenging and transformative work, but it is the most rewarding and enjoyable job you'll ever have. Now take a deep breath and turn the page as you open to a new chapter in your life.

Chapter 5

HEALING YOUR MIND

"The greatest discovery of any generation is that human beings can alter their lives by altering the attitudes of their minds."

ALBERT SCHWEITZER

COMPONENTS OF OPTIMAL MENTAL HEALTH

Peace of mind and contentment
- A job that you love doing
- Optimism
- A sense of humor
- Financial well-being
- Living your life vision
- The ability to express your creativity and talents
- The capacity to make healthy decisions

COMPONENTS OF OPTIMAL EMOTIONAL HEALTH

Self-acceptance and high self-esteem
- The capacity to identify, express, experience, and accept all of your feelings, both painful and joyful
- Awareness of the intimate connection between your physical and emotional bodies
- The ability to confront your greatest fears
- The fulfillment of your capacity to play
- Peak experiences on a regular basis

One of the most exciting developments in the field of medicine in recent decades has been the scientific verification that our physical health is directly influenced by our thoughts and emotions. The reverse is also true: Overwhelming evidence now exists showing that our physiology has a direct correlation to the ways we habitually think and feel. While Eastern systems of medicine, such as traditional Chinese medicine and Ayurveda, have for centuries recognized these facts and stressed the importance of a harmonious connection between body and mind, in the West this mind-body connection did not begin to be acknowledged until research conducted in the 1970s and '80s conclusively revealed the ability of thoughts, emotions, and attitudes to influence our bodies' immune functions. In fact, many of the scientists exploring this relatively new field of have concluded that *there is no separation between mind and body.*

In order to heal our minds and emotions, it helps to know what we mean by the term *mental health.* From the perspective of holistic medicine, the essence of mental health is peace of mind and feelings of contentment. Being mentally healthy means that you recognize the ways in which your thoughts, beliefs, mental imagery, and attitudes affect your well-being and limit or expand your ability to enjoy your life. It also means knowing that you always have choices about what you think and believe; are aware of your gifts; are practicing your special talents and working at a job that you enjoy; and are being clear about your priorities, values, and goals. People who have made a commitment to their mental health live their lives with rich reserves of humor and optimism. They have chosen a nurturing set of beliefs and attitudes that fill them with peace and hope. Most people who buy this book do so with the belief, however minimal, that they or a loved one will not have to take asthma medications for the rest of their lives and will free themselves of living with the fear of an asthma attack. Since you have read to this point and begun practicing the physical components of the Asthma Survival Program, your belief has probably been strengthened considerably. You can determine your own state of mental health by referring to the appropriate section of the

Wellness Self-Test at the end of Chapter 3, and then use the information in this chapter to improve the areas you may need to work on.

The term *mental health* can be interpreted to include not only our thoughts and beliefs but also our feelings. However, when your focus is specifically on "feelings," this is the realm of *emotional health*. These aspects of ourselves—**mental** and **emotional**—are for the most part inextricably related and together form the **mind** aspect of holistic health. As your healing journey progresses, you will increasingly come to recognize how your own distorted or illogical thoughts are the underlying cause of feelings such as anger, depression, anxiety, fear, and unfounded guilt. Learning how to free yourself from such distorted thinking patterns is the goal of this chapter, and of behavioral medicine, the aspect of holistic medicine that deals with this interconnectedness between physical, mental, and emotional health. Behavioral medicine includes professional treatment approaches such as *psychotherapy, mind-body medicine, guided imagery and visualization, biofeedback therapy, hypnotherapy, neurolinguistic programming (NLP), orthomolecular medicine* (the use of nutritional supplements to treat chronic mental disease), *flower essences,* and body-centered therapies like *Rolfing* and *Hellerwork*. However, with the exception of psychotherapy and hypnosis, the focus in this chapter is on proven self-care approaches that you can begin using immediately to heal the mind along with your dysfunctional lungs. They include *creating new beliefs and establishing clear goals, affirmations, breathwork, guided imagery, visualization, meditation, dreamwork, journaling,* and your approaches to both *work* and *play.* Each of these methods can help you become more aware of your habitual thoughts, attitudes, and emotions—both pleasurable and painful—in order to create a mind-set conducive to experiencing optimal health and more effectively meeting your professional goals and personal desires, including freeing yourself from the restraints of asthma.

THE BODY–MIND CONNECTION

Growing numbers of Western scientists and physicians now recognize that *body* and *mind* are not separate aspects of our being but interrelated expressions of the same experience. Their view is based on the findings of researchers working in the field of *psychoneuroimmunology (PNI),* also referred to as *neuroscience,* which for the past three decades has shown us that our thoughts, emotions, and attitudes can directly influence immune and hormone function. In light of such research, scientists now commonly speak of the mind's ability to control the body. In large part, this perspective is due to the scientific discovery of "messenger" molecules known as *neuropeptides,* chemicals that communicate our thoughts, emotions, attitudes, and beliefs to every cell in our body. In practical terms, this means that all of us are capable of both weakening or strengthening our immune system according to how we think and feel. Moreover, scientists have also proven that these messages can originate not only in the brain but from every cell in our body. As a result of such studies, scientists now conclude that the immune system actually functions as a "circulating nervous system" that is actively and acutely attuned to our every thought and emotion.

Among the discoveries that have occurred in the field of PNI are the following:

- Feelings of loss and self-rejection can diminish immune function and contribute to a number of chronic disease conditions, including heart attack.
- Feelings of exhilaration and joy produce measurable levels of a neuropeptide identical to interleukin-2, a powerful anticancer drug that costs many thousands of dollars per injection.
- Feelings of peace and calm produce a chemical very similar to Valium, a popular tranquillizer.
- Depressive states negatively impact the immune system and increase the likelihood of illness.

- Chronic grief or a sense of loss can increase the likelihood of cancer (and asthma—although this has not been scientifically documented, it is my clinical observation).
- Anxiety and fear can trigger high blood pressure.
- Feelings of hostility, grief, depression, hopelessness, and isolation greatly increase the risk of heart attack.
- Repressed anger is a factor in causing many chronic ailments, including sinusitis, bronchitis, headaches, and candidiasis.
- Acknowledgment and expression of feelings strengthen immune responses.
- Anger decreases immunoglobulin A (a protective antibody) in saliva, while caring, compassion, humor, and laughter increase it.
- Chronic stress has a broad suppressive effect on immunity, including the depression of natural killer cells, which attack cancer cells.

As exciting as these discoveries are, the studies that had the greatest impact on me were performed on multiple-personality patients at the National Institutes of Health (NIH). Scientists found that in one personality an individual could have the strongest possible skin reaction to an allergen or be severely nearsighted, but after shifting to another personality (an unconscious process in the *same* body) there was *no skin reaction* to the same allergen and perfectly normal *20/20 vision!* Science is just beginning to understand the depth and power of the connection between mind and body.

The implications of these discoveries are enormous and are producing a paradigmatic shift in physicians' approaches to treating chronic disease. They play an essential role in the Asthma Survival Program: If emotions and attitudes can contribute to causing heart disease and cancer, it isn't too difficult to appreciate how they can also play a role in asthma. They are also tremendously empowering for anyone committed to holistic health. Once you accept the fact that there is an ongoing, instant, and intimate communication occurring between your mind and your body via the mechanisms of neuropeptides, you can also see that the person best qualified to direct that communication in your own life is you. Learning how to do so effectively can enable you to become your own twenty-four-hour-a-day healer by becoming more conscious of your thoughts and emotions and managing them better to improve all areas of your health. The first step in this process is acknowledging that you can no longer afford to continue feeding yourself the same limiting messages you most likely have been conditioned to accept since early childhood. Scientists now estimate that the average person has approximately fifty thousand thoughts each day—yet 95 percent of them are the same as the ones he or she had the day before. Typically such thoughts are not only unconscious but often critical and limiting. For example, "I'll never be able to cure this asthma [or any chronic illness]." "I'll always be dependent on these inhalers." "I should've done _____ to have prevented this situation." "I can't realize my greatest potential or fully enjoy my life as long as I'm stuck with this condition." When you're hearing messages like these repeated many times during the course of a typical day, it's easy to understand why for most people with a chronic condition like asthma, *fear, anger, hopelessness, sadness,* and *depression* may become their predominant feelings. You've just read that these painful emotions can be associated with weakening the immune system while also contributing to a myriad of physical problems. Respiratory disease is no exception. However, *by consciously taking control of your thoughts and recognizing how they govern your behavior, you can dramatically change your life and heal your dis-ease.* You will gain the freedom to think, feel, and believe as you choose, thereby flooding your body's cells with positive, life-affirming messages capable of contributing to your optimal health.

5. PLAY/PASSION, MEANING/PURPOSE

The fifth item on my list of the *essential 8* is a mental/emotional (and spiritual/social) health practice focused on living a life filled with passion. This requires a level of self-awareness that will allow you to better understand and appreciate yourself while recognizing:

- your greatest talents and gifts
- what you most enjoy in life—what feels like play to you
- what would give your life greater meaning
- the purpose of your life—what you believe you came here to do

The next step on your path to optimal health is for you to begin creating a life that is more in accord with the responses to these self-posed questions. I've described this condition as the unlimited and unimpeded free flow of life force energy through your body, mind, and spirit. The remainder of this and the following chapter provide a variety of approaches to enhance this flow of life energy through your mind and spirit. They will provide you with valuable tools for gaining greater peace of mind, self-acceptance, and the self-esteem required to proceed on your healing path and enjoy more play and passion in your life.

PSYCHOTHERAPY

The field of psychotherapy, an outgrowth of the theories and discoveries of Sigmund Freud, continues to evolve more than a hundred years since its inception. In addition to the mental and emotional benefits commonly attributed to psychotherapy, a growing body of research has documented that physical benefits can also occur. For example, in a study conducted at the UCLA School of Medicine by the late Norman Cousins, a group of cancer patients receiving psychotherapy for ninety minutes a week showed dramatic improvement in their immune systems after only six weeks. During that same period the control group—other cancer patients who received no counseling—showed no change in immune function whatsoever.

Psychotherapy, by its very nature, is not a self-care protocol but can be extremely valuable for individuals struggling with deep-rooted mental and emotional problems. The most popular forms of psychotherapy are *classical* or *Freudian psychoanalysis, Jungian psychoanalysis, family therapy, cognitive/behavioral therapy, brief/solution-focused therapy,* and *humanistic/existential therapy.* Though they all share the same goal of helping patients achieve mental health, their approaches can vary widely.

If you feel that psychotherapy may help you, you will gain the most benefit by choosing the approach best suited to your specific needs and objectives. In addition, be aware that the work of psychotherapy is increasingly being conducted by nonpsychiatrists, including psychologists, social workers, and pastoral counselors. One of the reasons for this, perhaps, lies in the fact that many of today's patients seeing psychiatrists are given a psychiatric diagnosis (depression, manic-depressive, obsessive-compulsive, etc.) and then treated with drugs, such as the antidepressant Prozac. This trend within psychiatry, a move away from counseling and toward greater drug therapy, makes it a less desirable choice for someone interested in a holistic and self-care approach. While psychotherapeutic drugs can be effective at times, especially over the short term, each of the drugs commonly prescribed by psychiatrists has the potential to cause unpleasant side effects. Equally important, by focusing on treating psychological symptoms with drugs, many psychiatrists are depriving their patients of the opportunity to change their attitudes and behavior and to learn how to understand and grow from their emotional pain. Finally, whichever type of psychotherapist you choose, make sure that he or she is someone with whom you are comfortable. Psychotherapy can only be effective in a situation of trust, so you may wish to interview a number of therapists before making your choice.

BELIEFS, ATTITUDES, GOALS, AND AFFIRMATIONS

In his classic treatise *The Science of Mind,* noted spiritual teacher Ernest Holmes wrote: "Health and sickness are largely externalizations of our dominant mental and spiritual states. A normal healthy mind reflects itself in a healthy body, and conversely, an abnormal mental state expresses its corresponding condition in some physical condition." At the time Holmes wrote those words, in the mid–1920s, modern science was far behind him in understanding how *our thoughts directly influence our physical health.* But today a growing body of evidence not only verifies this fact but also indicates that it is our predominant, habitual beliefs that determine the thoughts we primarily think. Socrates stated that the unexamined life was not worth living. Based on today's research in the field of behavioral medicine, we may paraphrase his statement to say, *"The unexamined belief is not worth believing in."* Yet most of us have never taken the time to actually examine the beliefs we hold, and therefore remain unaware of how they may be influencing our well-being.

The importance of beliefs in the overall scheme of human functioning is confirmed by placebo studies. A placebo is a dummy medication or procedure possessing no therapeutic properties that works only because of our belief in it. Detailed analysis of thirteen placebo studies from 1940 to 1979, including 1,200 patients, found an 82 percent improvement resulting from the use of medications or procedures that subsequently proved to be placebos.

Changing your beliefs is essential to your success with the Asthma Survival Program. Many people suffering with asthma have been told by their physicians: "You're going to have to learn to live with this problem"; "The only thing that can be done is to take medication—anti-inflammatories and bronchodilators to control the symptoms"; "If you adhere to the established asthma management guidelines, you may eventually be able to take less medication"; or "There's nothing that can cure your asthma [or the majority of diseases]." These statements are, however, only beliefs. They are based on the limitations of modern medical science, a highly scientific and technologically advanced approach to the treatment of disease, and they are delivered to the patient by a highly educated individual in a society that defers to expertise. These pronouncements, which are in some cases death sentences, are quickly accepted by most patients and become a part of their own belief system. The vast majority of people with terminal diseases who accept whatever their doctors tell them (these patients are called "compliant") die very close to their predicted life expectancy. By contrast, patients who challenge their physician's "death sentence" tend to survive much longer, and some of them go on to achieve full recoveries. In *Love, Medicine, & Miracles,* Bernie Siegel, M.D., vividly describes how the beliefs and attitudes of many of his cancer patients affected the outcome of their disease.

Most of the beliefs held by Americans have been defined by the standards, or norms, of our society, but how well does the norm fit you, a unique individual? If all of us attempted to conform, the world would be a boring place, devoid of creativity and innovation. We certainly wouldn't be enjoying the ease of living that technology has provided us were it not for the adventurous few who deviated from the conventional belief system.

Unfortunately, in every culture there is great pressure to conform. It isn't easy, to say the least, to hold beliefs that run counter to prevalent attitudes. Society, friends, and family all tell us we have strayed with phrases such as "You should . . . ," "You ought to . . . ," or—if your belief has caused them a lot of discomfort—"You're crazy!" Most of the time we respond to this pressure by giving up our unreasonable, or even outrageous, beliefs. Ultimately almost all of us would prefer to be accepted and loved by others; besides, we tell ourselves, "It wasn't that big a deal anyway."

Your belief system has a profound impact on your life: what you eat and think; how you dress and behave; what you do for a living; whom you choose to marry, befriend, or live with; how you spend your leisure time; what your values and goals are; and how you define health and quality of life. It also determines the nature of the silent messages you give yourself every day. All of us talk to ourselves, and this internal dialogue has a great deal to do with our state of mental health. These messages may be generally self-critical ("You stupid . . ." "Why did I say that?" "Why did I do that?" "How could I . . . ?" "I should've [could've] . . ."); limiting ("I'll never be able to . . ."); or accepting and supportive ("Good job!" "That's fine." "I did the best I could."). Almost all of my patients are very hard on themselves. They are self-critical and put themselves under a great deal of unnecessary pressure, while at the same time most are high achievers. As human beings we are imperfect; all of us make mistakes. The way we respond to these failings is what creates more—or lessens—stress in our lives. Our pattern of response is one we probably have been repeating reflexively since childhood.

A very simple yet powerful exercise that can help you become more conscious of your thoughts, beliefs, and emotions is to devote fifteen minutes to writing out all that you are thinking during that time. Do this when you are not likely to be disturbed and don't edit anything out. After a few days of practicing this technique, many of your predominant beliefs will have been expressed on paper. Read them over. If they don't feel nurturing, build confidence and self-esteem, or regenerate you, clearly they are not serving you and need to be either eliminated or changed. Pay particular attention to the *shoulds*, *coulds*, and *nevers*. Before you discard what you write, examine your statements for possible clues to aspects of your life that may require more of your attention. For instance, if one of your statements reads, "I hate going to work," more than likely you may need to change your attitude about your job, or leave it for one that is more fulfilling and better suited to your talents. (If the thought of leaving your job raises the thought, "How will I provide for myself and my family?" realize that this in itself can be a limiting thought. Numerous options will become available to you once you liberate yourself from your old assumptions and beliefs.)

Once you have identified beliefs that are holding you back from your goals and desires or negatively impacting your health, the next step is to begin to *reprogram* your mind with thoughts, ideas, and images more aligned to what you want. One of the most effective ways to do this is through the use of **affirmations,** or positive thoughts that you repeat to yourself either verbally or in writing in order to produce a specific outcome. Affirmations are positive statements repeated frequently, always in the present tense, containing only positive words, and serve as a response to an often-heard negative message or as expression of a goal. For example, if some of the previous critical messages sound familiar to you, two affirmations that would help counteract them are "I love and approve of myself" and "I am always doing the best I can." These positive thoughts create images that directly affect the unconscious, shaping patterns of thought to direct behavior. In doing so, they act as powerful tools to unleash and stimulate the healing energy of love present in great abundance within each of us.

The purpose of affirmations is to replace habitual, limiting thought patterns and beliefs with more nurturing images of how you want your life to be. When affirmations are practiced regularly, they have the power to create optimal health by infusing the immune system with the life energy of *hope,* which triggers the activity of neuropeptides in the cells. Affirmations can be used to address virtually all aspects of your life, enhancing self-esteem, improving the quality of relationships, dealing with illness, and launching a more rewarding career.

Because of the simple nature of affirmations, the greatest challenge in using them is to suspend judgment long enough to allow them to produce the results you desire. When people begin repeating affirmations, they usually don't believe what they're saying (that's why they're saying them), although they would like to. Using affirmations is like reprogramming a computer. Your subconscious mind is the computer that has been receiving the same message for years—as the direct result of the thoughts and beliefs you have held for most, if not all, of your life. Now you are going to change the input with new "software."

Most computers have a total capacity for processing information far beyond the ability of the majority of computer operators to access it. Similarly, neuroscientists believe that the average person uses only 5 to 10 percent of his or her total brain capacity. As mentioned earlier, this average person has about fifty thousand thoughts every day, and it is estimated that 95 percent of them are the same ones he or she had the day before. Since your brain is hearing the same "program" repeated over and over again, it's no wonder you are able to realize only a small fraction of your (and your brain's) full potential. *Mental health will help to develop your creativity—you'll be re-creating yourself—while allowing you greater access to the parts of your brain that have been dormant.* It is in that recreational process that you'll find an almost limitless supply of joy and passion, along with some strong doses of pain to keep you on track.

The best time to say your affirmation is immediately following the negative message you repeatedly give yourself. When you're feeling the frustration of shortness of breath or wheezing and thinking to yourself, "This will never go away," you can follow that hopeless comment with the affirmation: "My lungs are healing and getting stronger every day." Positive statements like this while you're in the midst of practicing breathing exercises, changing your diet, taking the supplements, and the rest of the Asthma Survival Program, will not only help you to feel a little better, but will also increase your level of hope. And as your asthma improves, you'll believe the affirmation more and more until it is actually true.

After you read "Emotional Causes of Asthma" on page 224, think about how the information regarding some of the more common emotional factors might relate to you. At the same time, you should also consider the content of your often-heard silent messages. If you find that one or more of these specific issues applies to you, then I would recommend creating affirmations to help lessen the harmful impact they may be having on your lungs.

There are a variety of ways to use affirmations. Some people find they get their best results by writing each affirmation ten to twenty times a day. Others prefer to say them out loud, or to record them onto a cassette that they can then play to themselves daily. One powerful technique suggested by Louise Hay, author of the best-selling *You Can Heal Your Life* (see page 227), is to stare into a mirror and make eye contact with your reflection while verbally repeating each affirmation. Hay notes that this experience tends to bring up feelings of discomfort at first, and recommends that you continue the process until such feelings lessen or fade away altogether. You can experiment with these and other methods until you find the one that works best for you. Here are some other guidelines to ensure that you get the best results from your affirmation program:

1. **Always state your affirmation in the present tense and keep it positive.** For example, if one of your goals is to be free of job-related stress, the affirmation *I accomplish my daily responsibilities with ease and satisfaction* will produce far more effective results than statements such as *My job no longer makes me stressful.* The reason affirmations work is that the unconscious accepts them as statements of fact, and immediately begins to reorganize your life experience to match what you are telling it. So state *what you desire,* not what you wish to be free from, and write and say your affirmation in the present tense *as if your desire is already accomplished.*

2. Keep your affirmations short and simple, and no longer than two brief sentences.

3. Say or write each affirmation at least ten to twenty times each day.

4. Whenever you experience yourself thinking or hearing a habitual negative message, counteract it by focusing on your affirmation. Over time, you will find that your tendency to give yourself negative messages will diminish.

5. Schedule a time each day to do your affirmations and adhere to it. Doing something regularly at the same time each day adds to the momentum of what you are trying to achieve and eventually will become a positive, effortless habit.

6. Repeat your affirmations in the first, second, and third person, using your name in each variation. Using affirmations in the first person addresses the mental conditioning you have given yourself, while affirmations in the second and third person help to release the conditioning you may have been accepting from others. For example, if your name is Tom and one of your goals is to make more

money, you might write: *I, Tom, am earning enough money to satisfy all my needs and desires. You, Tom, are earning enough money to satisfy all your needs and desires. He, Tom, is earning enough money to satisfy all his needs and desires.* In each case, write out or repeat the affirmation ten times.

7. Make a commitment to practice your affirmations for at least sixty days or until you begin experiencing the result you desire.

You can use affirmations to help change any belief that doesn't feel good to you, to help you achieve any goal, or to create the life of your dreams. Most of my patients have come in because of one or more chronic physical or mental problems. Their objectives are clear: to stop living with chronic pain, to stop having sinus infections, to get rid of allergies or asthma, to have more energy, to suffer less anxiety, and so forth. After they have begun to see a definite improvement in their physical condition, which is usually after they have been working on the physical and environmentmal aspects of the specific holistic medical treatment program (Sinus, Asthma, or Arthritis Survival Program) for one to three months, I recommend that they create a "wish list" in the form of affirmations. The following is a powerful exercise for transforming your life and creating optimal mental health.

- **List your greatest talents and gifts.** You have several. These are things that are most special about you, or that you do better than most other people. Ask yourself, "What do I most appreciate about myself?"
- **Next, list the things you most enjoy**—both activities and states of being—for example, "I really enjoy just being in the mountains, or on a beach." There will be some overlap with your first list. Many of the activities you enjoy doing are the things you're best at.
- **Next, list the things that have the most meaning for you.** This is important, because if your goal doesn't meaningfully encompass more than one area of your life, or have

benefit to others in some way, more than likely it is incomplete, and you will lack the passion necessary to commit to it. As you list the meaningful things in your life, you will more easily recognize the talents and activities you enjoy that are most worth your while.

- **Now make a wish list of all your goals or objectives in every realm of your life**—physical/environmental, mental, emotional, social, and spiritual. Physical and environmental goals can include recovering from illnesses or ailments, engaging in or mastering a particular physical activity (anything you've ever considered doing), or living or working in a certain place. Mental goals might address career plans, financial objectives, and any limiting beliefs that you'd like to change. Emotional goals have to do with feelings and self-esteem. Social goals are about your relationships with other people, while spiritual objectives have to do with your relationship with God or Spirit. As you do this part of the exercise, ask yourself, "What does my ideal life look like?" "Where do I see myself five or ten years from now?" "What is my purpose—what am I here to do?" Do *not* give yourself a time frame within which to attain any of these goals, and remember, it is *not* necessary to have a plan for getting there.

- **Next, reword all of your goals into affirmations.** For example, a goal might be "I'd like to cure my asthma." Some simple affirmations might be: "My lungs are now completely healed" or "My breathing is improving every day." Then compile a list of about ten affirmations that address your most important goals and desires, and the most limiting beliefs or critical messages that you'd like to change. As you'll read in the following pages, many people with asthma have suppressed tears from grief, a lack of freedom, a lack of nurturing, unmet needs, and a fear of surviving. Effective affirmations for asthma might be *"It is safe for me to take charge of my own life." "I choose to be free." "I am meeting all of my greatest needs and desires." "I am loved and I am safe."*

- **Recite your entire list at least once a day, and whenever you hear a negative, limiting, or critical message,**

recite the one affirmation that corresponds to that message. Or you can record them onto a cassette and listen to them in your own voice. Perhaps the most effective method for deriving benefit from affirmations is to *write, recite,* and *visualize* them (see "Guided Imagery and Visualization" below). Using this method, you would write down your affirmation while reciting it aloud, and then close your eyes and imagine what the affirmation looks and/or feels like, engaging as many of your senses as possible. If you can't picture it, it helps to *feel* your affirmations as you recite or write them, since this brings more energy to the experience. Make the process as vivid and real as possible.

I learned this technique from a patient, a man who owns an oil company and works part-time as a psychotherapist. He'd had a terrible case of chronic sinusitis for many years. On our second session, one month into the Sinus Survival Program, I presented this idea of changing some of his limiting, critical, or negative beliefs and clarifying his goals and objectives as a foundation of greater mental health. Shortly after this visit, he formulated a lengthy list of affirmations and goals. Once each day he recited every one of his new beliefs, then wrote them down on a sheet of paper, and after each one he closed his eyes and visualized what that desire or goal would look or feel like. When I next saw him, just over two months later, he told me that he had been repeating this procedure of reciting, writing, and visualizing for sixty consecutive days. He was thrilled to report to me that at least half of his affirmations and goals had already become a reality, including healthy sinuses! He continues to practice this method (using new affirmations) along with the physical and environmental health recommendations that he had implemented at the outset of the program. It is now more than seven years since my third session with him. During that time he has had only two sinus infections, and his chronic sinusitis remains cured.

My patients' affirmation/goal lists provide a blueprint of our work together. The lists also become their personal vision and give direction to their own self-healing process.

You must be able to clarify your desires to have any chance of obtaining them, and as you do this exercise, try to be as specific as possible. The next step is to believe, however minimally, that it is possible for you to meet these goals. The more you repeat the affirmations, the stronger your belief will become.

The third step in this formula for self-realization is *expectation*. The stronger your belief and the more objectives you have already reached, the higher will be your level of expectation. After my chronic sinusitis was cured, I developed the belief that anything is possible, one that has helped me to realize other dreams. Whatever it is that you *desire*, as long as you *believe* it's possible, you can *expect* it to happen. It is not necessary to know how, or to have a definite plan. Just be patient and flexible and be willing to accept the result, even if the "package" in which it arrives is different from what you had envisioned. If your objectives are clear, your intuition will help you make the right decisions to get what you want. Remember that you can always choose what to believe. Rather than continuing with the attitude "I'll believe it when I see it," why not try "When I believe it, then I'll see it."

I've repeatedly seen this technique change lives in a variety of ways other than disease. My favorite example is a woman from Tennessee whom I was treating for chronic fatigue, allergies, and sinusitis. In the early years of my holistic practice, I worked with a number of patients long-distance over the phone, never actually meeting them in person. An R.N. in her fifties, she taught in a nursing school in a small town and had never married, although she wanted to. She had resisted putting marriage on her goal list because, as she explained to me, "I know all the eligible men in town and in my church, and there aren't any possible candidates." I convinced her to include it on her goal list, and her affirmation read simply: *I am happily married.* Within a few months, she received a letter from a former professor of hers with whom she had had a friendship years earlier. His wife had died the year before, and he wanted to visit his former student. Within months they were engaged, and a year after beginning her affirmation she was happily married. Her tears of joy over the phone and her gratitude left me in tears as well. We both felt as if we had experienced a miracle.

How you choose to see your asthma or any other chronic condition can play a vital role in the way the disease affects you and whether or not it goes away. Some of the early reactions to a chronic or life-threatening disease are denial ("There must be some mistake"), anger and frustration ("Why me?" "What terrible luck"), self-pity ("I'll never be able to enjoy life again"), and resignation ("I'll just have to put up with it and continue to live this way for the rest of my life"). All of these are quite normal and understandable responses to something as devastating as an incurable condition. However, if you are interested in healing yourself, it is important to get beyond this point and look at your disease in a different light. According to Bernie Siegel, who contributed the following material to the book *Chop Wood, Carry Water,* you have several choices:

- **Accept your illness.** Being resigned to an illness can be destructive and can allow the illness to run your life, but accepting it allows energy to be freed for other things in your life.
- **See the illness as a source of growth.** If you begin to grow psychologically in response to the loss the illness has created in your life, then you don't need to have a physical illness anymore.
- **View your illness as a positive redirection in your life.** This means that you don't have to judge anything that happens to you. If you get fired from a job, for example, assume that you are being redirected toward something else you are supposed to be doing. Your entire life changes when you say that something is just a redirection. You are then at peace. Everything is OK and you go on your way, knowing that the new direction is the one that is intrinsically right for you. After a while you begin to *feel* that this is true.

- **Death or recurrence of illness is no longer seen as synonymous with failure after the aforementioned steps are accomplished, but simply as further choices or steps.** If staying alive were your sole goal, you would have to be a failure because you do have to die someday. However, when you begin to accept the inevitability of death and see that you have only a limited time, you begin to realize that you might as well enjoy the present to the best of your ability.

- **Learn self-love and peace of mind, and the body responds.** Your body gets "live" or "energy" messages when you say "I love myself." That's not the ego talking, it's self-esteem. It's as if someone else is loving you, saying that you are a worthwhile person, believing in you, and telling you that you are here to give something to the world. When you do that, your immune system says, "This person likes living; let's fight for his or her life."

- **Don't make physical change your sole goal.** Seek peace of mind, acceptance, and forgiveness. Learn to love. In the process, the disease won't be totally overlooked—it will be seen as one of the problems you are having, and perhaps one of your fears. If you learn about hope, love, acceptance, forgiveness, and peace of mind, the disease may go away in the process.

- **Achieve immortality through love.** The only way you can live forever is to love somebody. Then you can really leave a gift behind. When you live that way, as many people with physical illnesses do, it is even possible to decide when you die. You can say, "Thank you, I've used my body to its limit. I have loved as much as I possibly can, and I'm leaving at two o'clock today." And you go. Then maybe you have spent half an hour dying and the rest of your life living; but when these things are not done, you may spend a lot of your life dying, and only a little living.

I realize that most of you will not die from your asthma, but each of these options for looking at physical illness can work for you as a form of preventive medicine. In my experience, chronic pain and imminent death have provided the greatest motivation for people to change, but why wait until you have reached that point of crisis?

EMOTIONAL CAUSES OF ASTHMA

Gerald Epstein, M.D., is an assistant clinical professor of psychiatry at Mt. Sinai Medical Center in New York City who has been engaged in PNI (psychoneuroimmunology) research under the auspices of the NIH Office of Complementary/Alternative Medicine for nearly a decade. As a result of his intensive work with asthmatics and mental imagery he believes that the emotional factors underlying asthma may be "a cry for freedom, or it may be about abandonment, loss, and/or dependency."

In my practice and that of Dr. Nelson, we have observed several consistent mental and emotional patterns in our asthmatic patients. Asthmatics are typically highly sensitive to disharmony in their physical, emotional, and social environment. They are often people with a diminished sense of freedom of expression as a result of a family dynamic in which they experience *enmeshment,* a smothering love, usually from their mother. They usually have a *lack of joy* resulting from an acute sense of loss. Their *grief* stems from *abandonment,* physical and/or emotional (usually from father); a lack of nurturing *touch* and *affection* as an infant or child; and the *absence of bonding between parents.*

In a ten-year study on asthmatics performed at the National Jewish Center for Immunology and Respiratory Medicine, they found that children in families that experienced intense levels of stress were three to four times more likely to develop asthma. The earlier in life the stress was experienced (even while the child was *in utero*), the greater the risk of asthma. We've seen that the stress results from both present familial relationships and past transgenerational bonding issues—that is, the inability to have intimate relationships between generations. These may manifest in the asthmatic child with feelings of melancholy and a sense of emptiness. This is particularly true when there is an absent father—either physically, emotionally, or both. The mother can either remain distant while experiencing her own feelings of abandonment, or make the child her "surrogate" for love and end up smothering him or her with excess attention. Parents who are not bonded with each other will have difficulty bonding with the child, especially with physical touch and affection. The behavioral and emotional environment created by the parents triggers feelings of internal chaos in the child that can result in a distrust and fear of their external emotional and social environment. Their unsuccessful attempts to bond with the adults closest to them increases feelings of fear of abandonment and possibly even fear of not surviving. Rather than a safe, joyful, positive experience of life, one in which they can "breathe in" fully and easily with those in their immediate environment, they have learned at an early age that their external environment is not entirely a happy, secure, or nurturing one.

The child's immune system can then become more reactive—more *allergic* to his or her environment. The primary function of the immune system is to discern between self and "not-self." On a deep, subconscious level the child feels acutely the disharmony in his environment and expresses this feeling through a repelling and heightened sensitivity to what is perceived as "not-self." This reaction results in large part from the assault on the child's innocence from unmet basic needs for nurturing. The lack of connection to one or both parents engenders a deep sense of grief, loss, and loneliness—a metaphor for the loss of connection to the breath of life. The toxic family relationships act like a virus, or a huge exposure to pollen, that assault the mucous membranes and trigger the immune system to mount an attack and throw off the perceived toxin. Wheezing, sneezing, runny nose, and coughing are all the body's attempts to remove an allergen, or a substance that is "not-self." The medical term for asthma—*reactive airway disease*—describes a heightened sensitivity in the mucous membranes of the lungs, which can be seen as metaphorically representing emotional reactivity to the family environment. The unconscious pathologic emotional process initially creates an attempt to stop the social disharmony that is failing to meet the child's basic needs (mild asthma), and may progress to more severe asthma requiring heroic acts of healing (emergency room visits with severe asthma attacks) to jolt the family out of its dysfunctional behavior to save the life of a family member. The act of joining together, even temporarily, for the sake of their child may result in more closeness between parents, mobilizing them to cooperate, put their personal needs aside, and rise to a higher purpose. The crisis makes caring for a severely asthmatic child an opportunity for the parents to respond to their child's need to experience a more tangible expression of love and bring them closer together as well. Perhaps asthma is simply a deep, unconscious, and dramatic way for the child to orchestrate a method for satisfying unmet needs. In his practice Dr. Nelson has witnessed several cases in which parents are coached to do affirmations with the child at night, with both parents present. They both offer touch and strokes, even during the child's first fifteen to twenty minutes of sleep. The focus of the affirmations is the parents' love and commitment to each other and to their child. When the affirmations are practiced consistently, the frequency and severity of the asthma attacks is significantly diminished.

Dr. Nelson is one of very few practitioners in the world who are highly skilled in the art of the Rayid Method of Personality Assessment. Although I've had only limited exposure to this modality, I've found Rayid to be an extremely valuable emotional health tool capable of identifying with impressive accuracy the emotional factors contributing to disease. The method involves reading the individual's genotype (personality traits) in the iris of the eye. The personality traits and unconscious emotions are presented and discussed with the patient, offering them another perspective on their illness and the healing lessons it may be providing them. The bulk of this section of the book has been derived from Todd Nelson's expertise in working with the Rayid Method and our collective clinical experience working holistically with asthma patients. The asthma pattern described above—the absence of nurturing, lack of touch, lack of bonding, inability to sustain joy, grief from loss, and fear resulting from survival needs being threatened—are all readily seen in the iris using the Rayid Method. Isn't it amazing that the patterning of the iris of the eye correlates so closely with the temperament of the patient?!

Chinese medicine has long recognized that asthma arises from imbalances in the lung meridian, which they associate with loss and grief. In their belief system this could be ancestral, not just limited to the present-generation family. Acupuncture can lessen this feeling and help free breathing.

Gaining a sense of being one's own authority, being in control, and authoring one's own life experiences is essential in healing asthma. For an adult, taking responsibility for creating one's own harmony is a critical component of the treatment program. Identifying your asthma triggers, many of which are toxic individuals, and establishing boundaries and more effective communication is extremely important. For children, it takes the mobilization of the entire family to create a loving, safe, intimate, nurturing environment so that the child can "breathe free." In this way, the asthmatic child provides the whole family with the opportunity to heal!

The book *Asthma Free in 21 Days, the Breakthrough MindBody Healing Program,* by Kathryn Shafer, Ph.D., and Fran Greenfield, M.A., outlines a wonderful series of breathing techniques, imagery, and affirmations they call the FUN program: Focus, Undo, Now act! This program is born out of Dr. Shafer's personal experience with asthma since the age of fifteen months. Dr. Shafer says, "[in asthma] the issue is *freedom*—freedom from smothering relationships, freedom to be oneself, freedom to choose, and freedom to enjoy and experience life!"

Louise Hay has written an excellent book on self-healing called *You Can Heal Your Life,* in which she focuses on the healing potential of affirmations as a means of learning to love yourself. Her book contains a list of medical conditions, each with the probable emotional cause and a corresponding affirmation. The emotional issues that she believes are most often associated with asthma are *smother love; inability to breathe for oneself; feeling stifled; suppressed crying.* The affirmations she recommends are:

"It is safe now for me to take charge of my life. I choose to be free. She suggests that parents of the asthmatic child use the affirmation "This child is safe and loved. This child is welcomed and nourished." In her book *Anatomy of the Spirit,* Carolyn Myss mentions that asthma is energetically related to the heart chakra. (In Ayurvedic medicine, there are seven primary *chakras,* or "spinning wheels," of bioenergy that comprise the basic structure of the emotional "body." Each chakra is associated with specific emotional energies.) The mental/emotional issues associated with the heart chakra and asthma are *love and hatred; grief and anger; resentment and bitterness; self-centeredness; loneliness and commitment; forgiveness and compassion; hope and trust.* Although all of the issues expressed by Louise and Carolyn may not relate to you, I have used both of their books as references for many years and have found them to be quite helpful and very often accurate.

I mentioned earlier that holistic medicine is based on the fundamental belief that unconditional love is life's most powerful healer—and its corollary, that all disease ultimately results from a deprivation of love. Multiple studies have demonstrated how powerfully love and intimacy can strengthen the immune system. When you consider the emotional factors contributing to asthma, and how significant they're proving to be, isn't asthma an excellent example of this holistic axiom? The lack of love, bonding, nurturing, freedom, as well as the experience of grief/loss, may help to explain not only the worldwide increase in the incidence of asthma, but possibly the profound discrepancy in who develops the disease. As I discussed in Chapter 2, the poorer black inner-city children are the most severely impacted population in the United States. The emotional factors that have been identified may apply to a significant portion of this group. But just the opposite is true for the rest of the world, where the more affluent children are more likely to suffer with asthma. Although I'm not certain, I would like to theorize about the following statistics that may be revealing a worldwide trend in emotional patterns of asthma. Perhaps the poorer East Germans living in highly polluted cities enjoy more closely knit families than do their more economically fortunate brethren in West Germany. Possibly the same is true in Zimbabwe, where the more affluent are 56 times more likely to develop asthma than are their financially deprived countrymen. One of the highest rates of asthma in children is in the United Kingdom (1 in 7), which may be one of the lowest-touch societies on the planet. Higher still is Australia (1 in 4) and New Zealand (1 in 3), both offspring of the unaffectionate British culture. Although both of these countries are also seriously impacted by the hole in the ozone layer, the United Kingdom is not, but it still ranks among the countries with the highest rates of asthma sufferers.

Obviously, asthma is a complex multifactorial condition with no simple explanation for its dramatic, nearly threefold increase over the past twenty years. But the emotional factors that are in the process of being identified are having a profound impact on this respiratory disease epidemic. Unless these causes are addressed and included as an integral part of the treatment program, asthma will remain an illness to be "managed," with only a slim hope for a cure.

GUIDED IMAGERY AND VISUALIZATION

Visualization is a skill all of us have and one that we use every day. Most of the time, however, we do so unconsciously, such as when we daydream. The fifty thousand thoughts we have each and every day are often accompanied by inner pictures, or imagery, with corresponding emotions. Since the 1970s, researchers, physicians, and other health care professionals have been examining how to harness these mental images in order to use them consciously to create improved states of well-being. Due to their continued work, thousands of individuals nationwide are learning how to use visualization and guided imagery to enhance their health. In many cases their results have been astounding. Since 1971, radiation oncologist O. Carl Simonton, M.D., for instance, has been a pioneer in developing imagery as a self-care tool for cancer patients to use to bolster their response rate to traditional cancer treatments, with remarkable success. The first patient to whom he taught his techniques was a 61-year-old man who had been diagnosed with a "hopeless" case of throat cancer. In conjunction with his radiation treatments, the man spent five to fifteen minutes three times a day imagining himself healthy. Within two months he was completely cancer-free.

A similarly remarkable case is that of Garrett Porter, a patient of Patricia Norris, Ph.D., another leader in the field of guided imagery. Garrett was 9 and had been diagnosed with an inoperable brain tumor. Using biofeedback techniques in conjunction with imagery based on Garrett's favorite TV show, *Star Trek* (he pictured missiles striking and destroying his tumor), Garrett was able to completely reverse his condition within a year, with brain scans confirming his tumor's disappearance.

Numerous studies also confirm the health benefits of imagery and visualization. For example, college volunteers who practiced imagery twice daily for six weeks experienced a marked increase in salivary immunoglobulin A as compared to a control group who did not practice imagery. In another study, the well-known drop in helper T-immune cells in students facing the stress of final examinations was greatly reduced in a group utilizing relaxation and imagery each day for a month before exams. And patients scheduled for gallbladder surgery who listened to imagery tapes before and after their operations had less wound inflammation, lower cortisone levels, and less anxiety than did controls who were treated with comparable periods of quiet only.

Like most of the other therapies outlined in this chapter, one of the most exciting things about guided imagery and visualization is that both techniques are powerful self-healing tools that can be used to create positive change in almost any area of your life. Besides physical health, imagery can help you feel more peaceful and relaxed, assist you in further developing your creative talents, create more fulfillment in your relationships, improve your ability to achieve career goals, and dissolve negative habit patterns. All that is necessary is a commitment to practice the techniques on a regular basis.

Guided imagery and visualization work to improve and maintain health because of their ability to directly affect our bodies at a cellular level, particularly with regard to neuropeptides. In addition, the use of imagery can often provide greater insight into causes and treatment for chronic conditions, guiding us toward the most personalized and effective solutions for our particular health problems. This occurs because our mental images are so deeply connected to our emotions, which, as we have discussed, are usually interconnected with the events in our lives. By using imagery, you can become better aware of what emotional issues may lie beneath the surface of your life and begin the process of healing them.

There are two types of guided imagery and visualization: preconceived or preselected images employed by you or your health care professional in order to address a specific problem and achieve a specific outcome, such as healing asthmatic lungs, and imagery that occurs spontaneously as you sit comfortably, eyes closed and breathing freely. Both forms have value, so try them both and see which works best for you. What follows are two techniques you can use to make imagery a part of your Asthma Survival Program. The first is a form of guided imagery, whereas the latter is conducive for allowing spontaneous imagery to occur on its own.

The Remembrance Technique. This exercise can be adapted to improve issues or conditions in any area of your life. It's called the Remembrance Technique because in our core selves we are already whole. In many respects, healing is simply a remembrance of that state in order to reconnect with it. Begin this exercise by sitting comfortably in a chair or lying down in bed. Select a time and place when you will not be disturbed. Close your eyes and focus on your breathing. Take a few deep, unforced breaths to help you relax. With each inhalation, imagine that soothing, relaxing energy is flowing through all areas of your body. As you exhale, visualize the cares and concerns of the day gradually disappearing. Do this for two or three minutes, allowing your breath to carry you to a place of calm relaxation.

Now choose the issue you want to focus on for the rest of the exercise, and recall a time when the outcome you desire was something you had already experienced. For example, if you have exercise-induced asthma, remember a time when you were in excellent health and could exercise strenuously without wheezing afterward. Allow yourself to reexperience that time, using all of your senses to make what you are imagining as vivid as possible. Once you have reconnected to the experience, bring it into the present *as if it were actually happening now.* Stay with the experience for at least five more minutes, mentally affirming that you *are* experiencing the state you desire here in the present.

Another form of preselected imagery is to focus on an image of healthy lungs, airways, and mucous membranes: a network of branching, wide-open tubes lined with a pink glistening membrane covered with thin clear mucus; as you picture this, you are taking deep belly breaths while visualizing the breath passing through the open airways and inflating your lungs on the inhale and deflating on the exhale. (To improve your ability to picture a normal healthy mucous membrane, look in the mirror and pull your lower lip down. The buccal mucosa lining your lip and cheeks resembles a healthy mucous membrane.) Prepare yourself in the same way I've described above—sitting, relaxed, and focused on breath. Even though this is a preselected image (like Garrett Porter's missiles striking his tumor), it can also be a dynamic process in which the image changes and evolves with each session of imagery. You might envision during one imagery session immune cells working feverishly to repair the surface of an inflamed (red) narrowed airway that is filled with thick mucus. As the imagery continues the membrane gradually becomes more pink, the thick mucus is thinned and markedly reduced in quantity, and the airway opens up, while the immune cells slow their pace and begin to relax on the surface of the membrane. Another time you might see a radiant white light filling every cell in the mucous membrane lining every bronchiole in your lungs, restoring it to perfect health with every in-halation you take. On exhalation, the debris containing toxins and allergens both within and on the surface of the cells is either expelled or disintegrated. Allow your imagery to be creative without placing any restrictions on it. There is no one correct image to use for healing asthma. Whatever works for you and feels good is the "right" image.

Spontaneous Imagery. In this exercise, instead of preselecting a specific outcome, you are going to allow your own unconscious to communicate with you through imagery about whatever situation in your life you choose to focus on. As in the preceding exercise, sit or lie down comfortably in a quiet place, close your eyes, and focus on your breath until you feel yourself settling into a deeper state of relaxation. Now focus on the physical problem you'd like to heal or the area in your life into which you desire to gain greater insight, allowing thoughts and images to freely and spontaneously emerge. Although you may have chosen your asthmatic lungs to focus on, you may be surprised by what you experience, but don't judge it. Trust that your un-conscious knows what you most need to understand, and allow your imagery to lead you to that answer. Continue this exercise for five to ten minutes, and when you complete it, write down what you experienced so that you can contemplate it for possi-ble further insight. As a variation to this exercise, you can first ask a question of yourself, such as "Why do I have asthma?" or "What do I have to learn from my asthma?" and then see what image appears. From there, you may find yourself engaged in a dialogue between yourself and your unconscious that results in answers and solutions you did not know were possible.

When you first begin to practice mental imagery techniques, don't be discouraged if at first "nothing seems to be happening." Like any new skill, achieving results in imagery takes time. Re-member that the language of your unconscious, like the sym-bolism of your dreams, is usually not literal or rational. It may take some time before you are able to grasp the messages of the images you perceive. Keeping a written log of your experience can make learning this new "language" easier.

HYPNOSIS, RELAXATON, AND BIOFEEDBACK

There are a number of studies documenting the therapeutic benefits (improved pulmonary function) of systematic *relaxation* training, *hypnosis,* and *biofeedback* with asthmatic patients. Although the latter two techniques can become effective self-care techniques, they require initial training from a highly skilled practitioner.

OPTIMISM AND HUMOR

In the Bible it is written: "A cheerful heart is good medicine, but a downcast spirit dries up the bones" (Proverbs 17:22). Science is now beginning to verify this ancient truth, revealing that optimism and humor are integral factors in one's overall health, providing both physical and mental benefits. One of the most famous anecdotes illustrating this point concerns Norman Cousins, who in his book *Anatomy of an Illness* attributed his recovery from ankylosing spondylitis (a potentially crippling arthritic condition of the spine) to the many hours he spent watching Marx Brothers movies and reruns of *Candid Camera* while taking megadoses of vitamin C. The more he laughed, the more his pain diminished, until eventually his illness completely disappeared, never to return. Based on his experience with humor, Cousins went on to explore mind-body medicine at UCLA. Today a number of institutions are studying the healing potential of humor, such as the appropriately named Gesundheit Institute in Arlington, Virginia, founded and directed by Patch Adams, M.D.

Some of the most in-depth research in this area has been conducted by Robert Ornstein, Ph.D., and David Sobel, M.D., who presented their findings in their book *Healthy Pleasures.* They discovered that the people who are optimally healthy also tend to be optimistic and happy, and possess the belief that things will work out no matter what their difficulties may be.

Such people maintain a vital sense of humor about life and enjoy a good laugh, often at their own expense. According to Ornstein and Sobel, they also expect good things of life, including being liked and respected by others, and experience pleasure in most of what they do. They usually look at stressful situations as temporary setbacks, specific to the immediate circumstance and due largely to external causes. Pessimists, on the other hand, when faced with life-challenging events, tend to think they will be permanent ("It's going to last forever"), generalize the problem to their whole lives ("It's going to spoil everything"), and blame themselves ("It's my fault"). Recent research at the Mayo Clinic suggests that pessimism is a significant risk factor for early death. Over 800 patients were given a personality test that categorized them as optimistic, mixed, or pessimistic. After their health status was evaluated thirty years later, the pessimists had a significantly higher-than-expected death rate.

Optimistic people also tend to laugh a lot, something that most likely plays an important role in their health. Studies have shown that laughter can strengthen the immune system. One study, for instance, found that test subjects who watched videotapes of the comedian Richard Pryor produced increased levels of antibodies in their saliva. Furthermore, subjects in the study who said they frequently used humor to cope with life stress had consistently higher baseline levels of those antibodies that help to combat infections such as colds.

Hearty laughter is actually a form of gentle exercise, or "inner jogging." Describing the physiological effects of laughter, Ornstein and Sobel write:

> A robust laugh gives the muscles of your face, shoulders, diaphragm, and abdomen a good workout. With convulsive or side-splitting laughter, even your arm and leg muscles come into play. Your heart rate and blood pressure temporarily rise, breathing becomes faster and deeper, and oxygen surges through your bloodstream. A vigorous laugh can burn up as many calories per hour as brisk walking or cycling.

The afterglow of a hearty laugh is positively relaxing. Blood pressure may temporarily fall, your muscles go limp, and you bask in a mild euphoria. Some researchers speculate that laughter triggers the release of endorphins, the brain's own opiates; this may account for the pain relief and euphoria that accompany laughter.

In short, laughter's benefits are many and profound. Unfortunately, most of us don't laugh enough. One recent study found that young children laugh about 400 times a day, while the average adult laughs only 14 times. When the question posed to octogenarians is "If you had your life to live over again, what would you do differently?" the answer often is "I'd take life much less seriously." Comedian George Burns, who lived to age 100, wrote the book *Wisdom of the 90's* at age 95. He attributed his ability to laugh at himself as well as loving what he did for a living as the most important factors in his longevity.

Both optimism and a sense of humor are directly related to our beliefs. If you wish to become more optimistic and experience more humor and fun in your life, practice the exercises outlined in this chapter. It may take time before you achieve the results you desire, but your commitment will prove well worth it and will impact your mood, mental health, and even survival. Nothing quite epitomizes the free flow of life force energy as laughter, and all of us can stand to laugh even more than we do. Be advised, however, that there is one side effect to this powerful form of self-healing: more pleasure.

EMOTIONAL HEALTH

The emotionally fit are able to identify their feelings and can express, fully experience, and accept them as well. I have heard contemporary American culture referred to as the "no-feeling" society. The feelings are certainly present, but as a result of our lifestyle we have constructed such formidable protective barriers around ourselves that to a great extent we have become unconscious of our feelings, especially the more uncomfortable ones.

Some people believe there are only two basic human emotions: love and fear. The so-called negative or painful emotions, such as anger, grief, anxiety, depression, envy, guilt, hatred, hostility, jealousy, loneliness, shame, and worry, are all expressions of fear. The feelings of acceptance, intimacy, joy, power, approval, and peacefulness are all aspects of love. The greater our degree of fear, the less capable we are of experiencing love.

With any chronic illness, including asthma, fear becomes the predominant emotion. When this occurs, your greatest liability is your *loss of love*—for yourself and those closest to you. It becomes a much greater challenge to nurture yourself and to feel fully alive when you're consumed with the anxiety and insecurity created by your ongoing physical discomfort and disability.

Some mental health professionals consider four basic emotions: love or joy, sadness, anger, and fear. So at any given moment you're feeling either glad, sad, mad, or scared, or some combination of these. In our culture it is not socially acceptable to express most of the "negative" emotions, and men especially are not supposed to show signs of weakness or insecurity or to cry ("Big boys don't cry"). The majority of us have learned to repress these feelings until we are unaware that we even have them. Society has helped us suppress our painful (negative) feelings by perpetuating the myth of an emotionally pain-free existence. The numerous ads in the media for analgesics to treat the pain of arthritis and headaches, and the common use of alcohol or drugs to dull the pain of an awkward social situation or personal crisis, give us the clear message that *not only is pain a bad thing, but life can be pain free.*

If we spend less time avoiding emotional pain, and instead focus our attention on it, accept it, and relax into it, the pain would diminish or even disappear. *If we continue to ignore and repress it, it often manifests itself as physical pain, illness, or disease.* Redford Williams, M.D., a researcher in behavioral medicine at the Duke University Medical Center, has gathered a wealth of data suggesting that chronic anger is so damaging to the body that it ranks with, or even exceeds, cigarette smoking, obesity, and a high-fat diet as a powerful risk factor for early death. Williams reported that people who scored high on a hostility scale as teenagers were much more likely than their more cheerful peers to have elevated cholesterol levels as adults, suggesting a link between unremitting anger and heart disease.

In another study, Dr. Mara Julius, an epidemiologist at the University of Michigan, analyzed the effects of chronic anger on women over a period of eighteen years. She found that women who had answered initial test questions with obvious signs of long-term, suppressed anger were three times more likely to have *died* during the study than those women who did not harbor such hostile feelings. Chronic sinusitis is usually associated with a tremendous amount of unexpressed anger, and I've also found it to be the primary trigger for most colds and sinus infections, as well as being an important contributing factor to arthritis and many other chronic conditions.

Clyde Reid is director of the Center for New Beginnings in Denver. In his insightful book *Celebrate the Temporary,* he says, "Leaning into life's pain can also be a lifestyle, and is far more satisfying than the avoidance style. It requires small doses of plain courage to look pain in the eye, but it prepares you for more serious pain when it comes. In the meantime, all the energy expended to avoid pain is now available for the business of living."

I am not advocating that you seek out painful experiences, nor am I proposing that you endure prolonged or persistent pain. That is called suffering. Health and happiness do not have prerequisites that require you to suffer. Life is to be enjoyed, but the notion that it can be lived entirely without painful feelings is an unhealthy belief. Pain and joy are intertwined, and **the more you allow yourself to accept, embrace, and feel both pain and joy, the greater will be your sense of emotional health.**

Of the mental-emotional connection, Albert Ellis, a psychologist and founder of the Institute for Rational-Emotive Therapy in New York City, has said that "virtually all 'emotionally disturbed' individuals actually think crookedly, magically, dogmatically, and unrealistically." David D. Burns, M.D., a psychiatrist and author of *The Feeling Good Handbook,* writes:

> Certain kinds of negative thoughts make people unhappy. In fact, I believe that unhealthy, negative emotions—depression, anxiety, excessive anger, inappropriate guilt, etc.—are *always* caused by illogical, distorted thoughts, even if those thoughts may seem absolutely valid at the time. By learning to look at things more realistically, by getting rid of your distorted thinking patterns, you can break out of a bad mood, often in a short period of time, without having to rely on medication or prolonged psychotherapy.

Burns offers the following list of thought distortions:

- **All-or-nothing thinking.** You classify things into absolute, black-and-white categories.
- **Overgeneralization.** You view a single negative situation as a never-ending pattern of defeat.
- **Mental filtering.** You dwell on negatives and overlook positives.
- **Discounting the positive.** You insist your accomplishments or positive qualities "don't count."
- **Magnification or minimization.** You blow things out of proportion or shrink their importance inappropriately.
- **Making *should* statements.** You criticize yourself and others by using the terms *should, shouldn't, must, ought,* and *have to.*
- **Emotional reasoning.** You reason from how you feel. If you feel like an idiot, you assume you must be one. If you don't feel like doing something, you put it off.
- **Jumping to conclusions.** You "mind-read," assuming, without definite evidence of it, that people are reacting negatively to you. Or you "fortune-tell," arbitrarily predicting bad outcomes.

- **Labeling.** You identify with your shortcomings. Instead of saying, "I made a mistake," you tell yourself, "I'm such a jerk . . . a real loser."
- **Personalization and blame.** You blame yourself for something you weren't entirely responsible for, or you blame others and ignore the impact of your own attitudes or behavior.

As I've already said, negative thoughts and the feelings they engender contribute to physical illness. The lack of control, fear of surviving, and the lack of joy and freedom experienced by many people with asthma are frequently associated with several of the above thought distortions. These repeated thoughts will often trigger anger (ultimately with ourselves) and depression (almost always fueled by repressed anger), which, if not expressed, can further diminish immune function and aggravate asthma. Many of these same critical and limiting messages are also preventing you from achieving your goals and seeing your "wish list" become a reality. These theories of Drs. Ellis and Burns constitute the foundation of cognitive psychotherapy—the form of counseling I've found to be highly effective for my patients.

One self-care approach you might try for gaining greater self-awareness is to attempt to identify the mental and emotional issues that may have contributed to causing your asthma. A method I've used with my patients for many years is to consider the possible benefits or secondary gain resulting from having this condition. They may not be readily apparent, but if you're open to this introspective exploration you'll usually find some answers, however minimal, to the question "What are the benefits of having asthma?" As I've previously mentioned, a child's asthma may help to bring the family together and fulfill his unmet needs for nurturing. But are these benefits still valid for you as an adult? Other possible gains may include "My husband [or wife] pays more attention to me"; "I don't have to work or exercise as hard"; "I'm no longer expected to perform at the level I had been, and that has reduced a lot of pressure [stress] that I'd been feeling." Whether it's more attention, a need to be cared for, job dissatisfaction, performance anxiety, or some other unmet need, I believe there are almost always some secondary gains associated with every chronic disease. Since you did not respond preventively, in order to meet those unconscious needs, your body created an illness. If these not-so-subtle benefits can be understood and you become more aware of what your needs and desires are, it will help considerably in identifying the emotional causes of your physical problem and allow you to work on resolving them. Once you have become aware of the issues, you can then begin expressing your emotions while addressing the unmet needs your feelings have revealed. The process continues with acceptance: knowing that it's okay to feel whatever you're feeling. This healing process will not only lead you to emotional health, it will help you practice preventive medicine, and will also take you a giant step closer to being free of your reactive airway dis-ease. Remember, a basic tenet of mind body medicine is that *your core issues are held in your tissues.*

BREATHWORK AND MEDITATION

The benefits of learning to breathe properly and consciously (see "breathing exercises," page 87) go far beyond the physical. Proper breathing can also improve your mood, make you mentally more alert, and help you to become more aware of deeply held and often painful feelings. Most important, by working with your breathing, you can begin to heal the wounded, rejected, unacknowledged, and disowned parts of yourself and bring them into wholeness.

The primary reason so many of us breathe unconsciously and inefficiently lies in the fact that our breathing process began traumatically at birth. We were forcibly expelled from the security of the womb and compelled to take our first breath on our own when we encountered the outside world. Often that first breath came as a harsh and unexpected shock, accompanied by pain and confusion. In order to suppress such pain, newborns typically follow their first inhalation by pausing and holding their breath for a moment as they struggle to make sense of their new environment. Today a number of researchers in the field of mental health speculate that this first pause in our breath not only sets the stage for a lifetime of shallow, inefficient breathing but also conditions us to suppress our painful emotions instead of learning how to accept and relax into them. You can observe this pattern in yourself the next time you find yourself feeling shock, fear, pain, or worry. If you take a moment to observe yourself in the initial experience of such emotions, more than likely you will find that you are also holding your breath or breathing very shallowly, or perhaps even wheezing.

Breathwork, also known as "breath therapy," is a means of learning how to breathe consciously and fully in order to deal with emotional pain more effectively and healthfully. There are many approaches to breathwork, ranging from ancient breathing techniques found in the traditions of *yoga, tai chi,* and *qi gong,* to modern-day methods such as *rebirthing* (also known as *conscious connected breathing*), developed by Leonard Orr, and *holotropic breathwork,* developed by Stanislav Grof. All of them have in common a focus on the breath and the ability to move energy through the body and connect you with suppressed emotions and limiting beliefs in order to heal them.

Most breathwork therapies use the technique of connected breathing, first pioneered by Leonard Orr. In connected breathing, each inhalation immediately follows the exhalation of the preceding breath without pause. (Typically we breathe unconsciously, pausing between inhalation and exhalation.) The pattern of respiration can vary according to technique. Sometimes it is rapid; sometimes it is deep, slow, and full. In addition, some approaches recommend breathing in and out through the mouth, instead of the nose, and both abdominal and chest breathing can be used. In rebirthing, sometimes the therapy is performed in a tub or underwater with the use of a snorkel, although this usually does not occur until after the client has had a number of "dry" connected breathing sessions and has become comfortable with the movement of energy and integration of emotions that commonly occur during the rebirthing process. (*Note:* I would not recommend rebirthing for an asthmatic, since it may aggravate the condition. However if you do try it, use the same precautions as you would prior to exercise.) Because of the emotional release that can result from breathwork, it is advisable to learn the techniques under the direction of a skilled breath therapist. Once you gain proficiency, however, you will have at your disposal a powerful self-healing technique that you can practice daily on your own.

Meditation also offers a multitude of emotional health benefits. There are numerous meditation techniques, but all of them can be accurately described as conscious breathing methods. Meditation's many physiological benefits include improved immune function; reduced stress, including decreased levels of adrenaline, cortisone, and free radicals; increased oxygen intake; relief from chronic pain and headache; lower blood pressure and heart rate; and a reduction of core body temperature, which has been linked to increased longevity. Among the psychological benefits of meditation are greater relaxation; improved focus on the present instead of regrets and worries about the past and future; enhanced creativity and cognitive functioning; heightened spiritual awareness (including insights leading to the healing of past emotional trauma); improved awareness and management of beliefs and emotions; and a greater compassion and recognition of others and oneself as parts of a greater whole.

The following is a simple meditation technique that utilizes breathing to promote mental calm. Select a quiet place and sit in a chair with your back straight and your feet on the floor. Close your eyes and begin abdominal or belly breathing, inhaling and exhaling through your nose at a rate of three to four full breaths (inhale and exhale) per minute. (This is the same rate recommended for the breathing exercises on page 87.) The object of this exercise is to stay focused on your breath, allowing whatever thoughts you have to come and go without being absorbed by them. Should you find your attention wandering, bring it back to your breath. You can also enhance the process by silently repeating a short affirmation, or a positive phrase, such as *God, love,* or *peace,* on both the inhale and the exhale. At first, try to do this exercise for five minutes once or twice a day, gradually working up to twenty minutes twice daily. You can use it in place of, or in addition to, your breathing exercises. Don't be discouraged if at first you find this exercise difficult to practice. For most Americans, sitting and breathing without thinking or external stimulation is not easy. With time and continued practice, especially in the morning and before you go to bed, you will begin to notice the benefits meditation affords. (For more on meditation, see Chapter 6.)

DEALING WITH ANGER

Unexpressed anger, or anger that is expressed inappropriately, is both harmful and extremely common in our society. Most of us were taught very early in life that anger was an unacceptable emotion. When it was expressed, it often elicited fear in us, and was usually equated with bodily harm and loss of control ("He's really lost it"; "He's out of control"). This inability to safely express anger has been shown to produce many serious health consequences, from heart attacks to sinus infections. Today many psychotherapists are combining sound and body movement techniques to help their patients deal with their anger, finding that such approaches can be far more effective than simply talking about it. The following techniques can be safely employed by anyone to release the highly charged emotional energy of anger. They are most effective when employed regularly as preventive measures, instead of allowing anger to build up into a state of chronic, health-impacting tension, much less explosive rage.

Screaming This is the most common anger-release technique, because all of us already know how to do it. In his novel *Tai Pan,* author James Clavell wrote that the chieftains of ancient Scotland for centuries maintained the custom of "the screaming tree." From the time they entered adolescence, males of the clan were instructed to go into the forest and select a tree to which they could express their discontent. Then, whenever their troubles grew too great to otherwise deal with, they would go to the forest alone and scream with the tree as their witness until their emotions settled.

The value of screaming is no secret to young children, who commonly scream when they are greatly upset, only to exhibit a smiling face moments afterward. For adults, the biggest difficulty involved is finding a place to scream in privacy. Screaming when you are home alone, in the basement or closet, in the car with the windows up, or in a secluded spot outside are all possibilities. To get the most benefit, take a deep abdominal breath before you scream, then direct the scream from your diaphragm or deep within your chest cavity, as this will protect your vocal cords. As you scream, slowly move your upper body from side to side or up and down. Usually, after two or three screams in succession, you will begin to feel much better. (*Note:* It's possible, although unusual, that screaming could trigger asthma. If you keep the screaming sessions brief, there should be no problem.)

The angry letter (not sent) This technique is increasingly employed by therapists to help their clients release their anger. It involves writing a letter to the person with whom you are angry, listing all of the reasons why you are upset with them. As you write, allow yourself to express whatever comes to mind, no matter how harsh or offensive it may seem. Once the letter is written, read it over, and if anything else occurs to you that you wish to express, write that down too before signing it. Then either burn the letter or tear it up into small pieces.

Punching Punching a bag, pillow, or sofa is another effective method of dissipating anger. Remember to grunt or yell with each punch. A variation of this method is to take hold of a pillow and hit it against the floor, sofa, or wall. With either approach, it takes only a few moments before you will start to feel your anger transforming into satisfaction and even joy. Remember, anger, in and of itself, is not a negative emotion to be shunned. It's only when it remains bottled up inside of us unex-

pressed that it becomes unhealthy. *Safely and appropriately expressing your anger in socially acceptable ways can dramatically improve the
way you feel, both emotionally and physically.*

However, simply venting anger doesn't do the whole job. In
fact, one study in April 1999 concluded that punching to release
anger actually tends to increase and prolong feelings of hostility.
Although this finding runs counter to my personal experience
and that of many of my patients who have benefited from this
practice, there are several additional steps that can be taken to release anger. You can start by recognizing that your anger may be
the result of unreasonable or even irrational demands you've
made on yourself or someone else, and that by maintaining
these demands you are hurting yourself with increased stress. It
is therefore in your best interest to release the demands and let
go of the anger.

Aerobic exercise This is another quick-fix method for dissipating anger and opening your nose and sinuses. However, if
you're especially enraged about a particular incident or situation,
wait at least twenty minutes and take some deep breaths before
beginning a strenuous workout. There can be a greater risk of
heart attack associated with exercise *immediately* following emotional trauma. Journaling, which I'll discuss in the next section,
is also an effective means of releasing anger but is not quite as
fast as punching and exercise.

DREAMWORK AND JOURNALING

Dreams can play an important role in your healing journey.
Serving as symbolic expressions of your inner emotional life,
dreams often provide the clues you need to better understand
your mental and emotional states, as well as the guidance you
may need to heal personal life situations. Dreams can also sometimes reveal how to heal physical disease conditions. This was illustrated in a dream of Alexander the Great recounted in Pliny's
Natural History. One of Alexander's friends, Ptolemaus, was dy-

ing of a poisoned wound, when Alexander dreamed of a dragon holding a plant in its mouth. The dragon said that the plant was the key to curing Ptolemaus. Upon awakening, Alexander dispatched soldiers to the place he had seen in his dream. They returned with the plant and, as the dream had predicted, Ptolemaus, as well as many others of Alexander's troops suffering from similar wounds, was cured.

In American society, dreams are often overlooked or ignored, although researchers like Stephen LaBarge, Ph.D., have in recent decades done much to scientifically demonstrate their importance. The two biggest obstacles that prevent us from getting the most benefit from our dreams are that we either do not remember or quickly forget them, or we do not know how to interpret the symbolism and imagery that dreams contain. Dream recall is a skill that anyone can develop with time and practice, however. One of the keys to dreamwork is to commit to focusing attention on your dreams. A deceptively simple way to do this is to tell yourself each night before you fall asleep that when you awaken you will remember what you dreamed during the night. At first you may not experience much success, but regular affirmation of this technique will instruct your unconscious to eventually make your dreams recallable.

As you start to remember your dreams, keep a pad and pencil or a tape recorder by your bed so that you can either write down or verbally record them immediately after you awaken. All of us dream an average of three or four times each night. With practice, many people who make the commitment to record and study their dreams are able to train themselves to spontaneously awaken after each dream cycle to record the gist of their dreams before settling back to sleep. Recording your dreams *immediately* after you awaken provides the best results, since dreams are quickly forgotten once you get out of bed and begin your day. Initially, all you may recall are fragments of your dream experience. Don't be discouraged if this is the case. Over time, the regular recording of your dreams will begin to yield more details. In addition, after you have recorded your dreams for a few weeks or months, as you read over your dream diary, you will start to notice how certain symbols and events tend to recur. Pay attention to such common themes: Usually they contain the most important messages that your dreams have for you.

Learning how to interpret the symbolism of your dreams takes time and practice. Certain psychotherapists, especially those with a background in Jungian theory, are skilled in dream interpretation and can help you, and a number of books on the subject can also guide you. Bear in mind, however, that your dreams are highly personal, and although many dream symbols do seem to be common to what Jung called "the collective unconscious," there is no such thing as a standard for dream interpretation that will work for everyone. As the dreamer of your own life, you are ultimately the person best suited to appreciate your dreams and discern their deepest meanings. By taking the time to do so, you can improve your mental and emotional health immeasurably.

Journaling is another simple but very effective way to become more conscious of your mental and emotional life and to help you better express your feelings. The practice of journaling entails keeping a written record of your thoughts, emotions, and any other daily experiences that you would like to better understand. Instead of recording your dreams, you will be keeping a journal of your waking activities. When journaling is done on a regular basis, it usually results in increased self-knowledge, often with insights that are both enlightening and enlivening. In a very real sense, journaling can help you become your own therapist or best friend: Instead of trying to express what you're feeling to someone else, through the process of journaling you tell it to yourself. The result is that your journal becomes your own emotional diary.

Many people who begin the practice of journaling are amazed to discover how the simple act of writing out one's daily experiences can lead to sudden or deeper insights into what they are feeling. Journaling can also help you become better aware of your beliefs, providing you with the opportunity to recognize and change those that may be limiting you. As you journal you will also start to take more control over what you are thinking and feeling, becoming less reactive to your life experiences and more creative in your approaches to dealing with them. Journaling also makes communicating with yourself easier and allows greater clarity, since you are free from judgment or criticism from others. Your journal is for you alone and isn't meant to be shared. Nor do you have to worry about spelling or grammar.

A number of researchers, including James W. Pennebaker, Ph.D., author of the book *Opening Up,* have documented the benefits that journaling can provide by writing about upsetting or traumatic experiences. For people who have difficulty expressing their emotions, particularly those that are judged to be negative, such as anger or fear, journaling can be especially valuable as a tool for self-healing. The results of a recent study measuring the effects of writing about stressful experiences on symptom reduction in patients with mild to moderate asthma and arthritis were published in *JAMA* in April 1999. The subjects in the study were asked to write about the most stressful event of their lives for twenty minutes for three consecutive days. They changed *nothing else* in their treatment regimen. Four months later, researchers found a marked improvement in lung function in the asthmatics and a significant reduction in the severity of disease in the arthritics. This landmark study is a clear demonstration of the therapeutic value of expressing emotions in treating a physical condition. Since most patients with asthma don't have the opportunity to relate their feelings to their physician, writing in a journal or writing unsent letters can be a highly effective self-care technique.

For best results, try to write in your journal around the same time each day. This will help you make journaling a healthy habit. Just before you go to bed can be an ideal time for journaling. You can express the emotions that you've been containing all day and can provide resolution to the day's events prior to going to sleep. Journaling and dreamwork will not only help you to heal mentally and emotionally (and physically) but can also open up new vistas of adventure that can last you a lifetime.

WORK AND PLAY

Do you enjoy your job? Does your work utilize your greatest talents? Is your job fulfilling and challenging? Sadly, for the majority of Americans the answer to these questions is no. Recent studies reveal that an alarmingly high proportion of our society—nearly 70 percent of us—do not experience satisfaction from our jobs. Unfortunately, there is a significant price to be paid for not loving your work, both physiologically and psychologically. For example, in a study conducted by the Massachusetts Department of Health in the late 1980s, it was found that the two greatest risk factors for heart disease lie in one's self-happiness rating and level of job satisfaction. Low scores in these two areas were shown to be better indicators of the likelihood for developing heart disease than are high cholesterol, high blood pressure, overweight, and a sedentary lifestyle. No wonder, then, that in the United States more heart attacks occur on Monday morning around nine o'clock than at any other time of the week.

Your job is a vital aspect of your mental health. If you find yourself working at a job that you do not enjoy, chances are that you continue to do so because of one or more of the following limiting beliefs: *I don't have a choice. I need the money. I'll never be able to make enough money doing what I love. I have no idea what I'd enjoy doing or what my greatest talents are.* By using the techniques outlined in this chapter, especially in the section "Beliefs, Attitudes, Goals, and Affirmations," you can begin to liberate yourself from these unhealthy beliefs. You'll discover that you are not bound to your job for life and you do have the ability to find a job for which you are better suited and that is more fulfilling. Every one of us is blessed with at least one God-given talent, and there is at least one activity that we enjoy doing that we do quite well. *That* is where you need to begin to investigate what your gifts are. Write down your talents as outlined in the goal-setting section above, followed by a list of activities you truly enjoy. Then brainstorm all the possible ways you can think of in which you can earn a living combining your talents with each of the activities you wrote down. List every idea that occurs to you, regardless of how ridiculous it may seem. As you continue to practice this exercise, you will have a much clearer idea of new job options. At the same time, acknowledge that you are seeking a greater level of fulfillment, are willing to change and take a risk, and are committed to begin the exploration that will lead you to work that you love doing. In the process, you may discover that your capabilities are limitless.

Even if you are fortunate to have a job you do enjoy, you may still be prey to another modern-day dis-ease: **workaholism.** According to the Economic Policy Institute in Washington, D.C., the majority of Americans are working longer and harder than they used to (the average work week is currently forty-six hours). Our yearly workload has increased by 158 hours, compared to that of twenty years ago, including longer commuting times, fewer paid holidays, and less vacation time. That's the equivalent of almost an extra month's work per year. To counter this tendency, it is essential that you regularly engage in the counterbalance to work: *play.*

Many of us have unfortunately relegated play to childhood; yet play is a crucial aspect of mental health and is unrivaled as a means of expressing joy, passion, exhilaration, even ecstasy. The word *play* comes from the Middle Dutch *pleyen,* which means "to dance, leap for joy, and rejoice," all activities that suggest a vibrantly healthy mental state. Play has also been defined as any activity in which you lose track of time. Believing that play is not appropriate adult behavior is both limiting and unhealthy.

If your work involves your greatest talents and is something you truly enjoy doing, work and play for you can seem virtually indistinguishable. Even so, to optimize mental health, find at least one other activity to participate in, besides your work, that you can thoroughly enjoy. Such activities include sports, games, dance, and creative pursuits such as playing a musical instrument, acting, singing, painting, crafts, and gardening. Although many people derive great pleasure from playing cards, chess, and other board games, or stamp or coin collecting, all of these are mental pursuits. To create a healthier balance, select activities that utilize your body, allow you to better express your feelings and creativity, and perhaps even bring you to a greater level of spiritual attunement. Ideally, the activity should be something so consuming and absorbing that it requires your total attention, providing a pleasurable escape from your normal tension, stress, and habitual thought patterns. Choose something that instinctively appeals to you and do it on a regular basis, for at least an hour three times a week. Be prepared to make mistakes and look silly. That's part of the risk—and the excitement—of doing something new. The more you commit to and practice whatever activity you choose, the better you'll become at it and the more you'll enjoy the benefits it provides.

We live in a society where work has become the greatest addiction, and the majority of us gauge our self-worth according to our achievements and net worth. For this reason alone the importance of play cannot be overemphasized. All of us, for a short time at least, need to regularly let go of that responsible, mature, working adult part of ourselves to reconnect with our woefully neglected playful "inner child."

SUMMARY

The biggest obstacles each of us must overcome to achieve optimal mental and emotional health are our largely unconscious denial and repression of emotional pain, and our limiting thoughts, beliefs, and attitudes, which combined create our unhealthy behaviors. The tools in this chapter will enable you to heighten your awareness, allowing you to consciously transform your life in harmony with your greatest needs and desires. The more you practice the methods outlined here, the more profound the impact you will have on your mental and emotional health, as well as your physical health and your asthma. *You will become more conscious of your behavior and gain the freedom to choose how you wish to think, feel, and behave.* By letting go of your fear of experiencing life more fully, you can **breathe freely** while embracing and accepting all of your thoughts, beliefs, and emotions. This will allow you the joy of realizing your life's goals and the exhilaration of the unimpeded free flow of life-force energy. Remember, only through fully experiencing *both pain and joy* can you truly use your unique gifts and talents to thrive and fulfill your life purpose. And *if you can't feel it, you can't heal it.* This holds true for asthma, arthritis, sinusitis, heart problems, and any other chronic dis-ease. Your underlying emotional pain will be mirrored back to you with the ill health of your body and/or your mind. But so, too, will vitality and happiness reflect a condition of radiant health.

Chapter 6

HEALING YOUR SPIRIT

"What profit does a man receive if he gains the whole world only to lose his soul?"

MATTHEW 16:26

COMPONENTS OF OPTIMAL SPIRITUAL HEALTH

Experience of unconditional love/absence of fear
- Soul awareness and a personal relationship with God or Spirit
- Trusting your intuition and a willingness to change
- Gratitude
- Creating a sacred space on a regular basis through prayer, meditation, walking in nature, observing a Sabbath day, or other rituals
- Sense of purpose
- Being present in every moment

The ultimate outcome of healing ourselves holistically is the recognition that we are truly spiritual beings, and the heightened awareness of the transcendent power known as God or Spirit. By making the commitment to become spiritually healthy, we open ourselves to the underlying life-force energy to which all religions refer and which is known in holistic medicine as *unconditional love*. Learning to love yourself in body, mind, and spirit is also the simplest and most direct way to learn to love God. To heal yourself spiritually means developing a relationship with Spirit in your own life and attuning yourself to

Its guidance in all aspects of your daily existence. By doing so, you will begin to experience a profound reduction in your feelings of fear, and a greater capacity for loving yourself and others unconditionally. You will also become better able to identify your special talents and gifts and use them to fulfill your life's purpose *while fully experiencing the power of the present moment.*

In the deepest sense, all *dis-ease* can be seen as a disconnection between ourselves and Spirit, and a deprivation of love. From that perspective, spiritual health encompasses not only a conscious awareness of the Divine but also an intimate connection to ourselves, our families, our friends, and our communities. Just as mental health encompasses emotional health, spiritual health embraces social health. You cannot have one without the other. This truth is illustrated in the lives of the world's great spiritual teachers, including Moses, Jesus, Mohammed, Krishna, and Buddha, all of whom remained closely connected to their communities throughout the course of their ministries. Despite the apparent differences in their instructions to us, at their core their messages are actually the same: *Place God first in all that you do, and love your neighbor as you love yourself.* As you reclaim your spiritual health, you fulfill their intention.

ACCESSING SPIRIT

"Every advance in knowledge brings us face-to-face with the mystery of our own being." MAX PLANCK, father of quantum physics

You may believe that you are incapable of experiencing Spirit in your life, but that is not the case. *Spirit is present in any moment when we feel profoundly alive.* During these special moments, our predominant emotions are exhilaration and joy. The late Jesuit priest and scientist Teilhard de Chardin described *joy* as "the most infallible sign of the presence of God." Usually these fleeting moments surprise us: Our perception of reality is suddenly free of our normal judgments and concerns. Time seems to slow as we lose ourselves in *pure awareness.* Examples of these moments include experiencing the birth of your child, time spent with your beloved, being present at the death of someone you love, witnessing a sunset, entering "the zone" while playing sports, and being in the presence of inspirational works of art. Such peak experiences can also occur unexpectedly and spontaneously during the course of your normal routine, sparked by something as innocuous as hearing your favorite song on the radio. For most of us, these moments may seem to be accidental occurrences.

The purpose of this chapter is to help make your encounters with Spirit a more frequent and conscious part of your life. As you learn to master the techniques that follow, recognize that Spirit operates in much the same fashion as do subatomic particles: Both can be identified without being directly observed. Most often, and especially at the beginning of your spiritual journey, Spirit will be identified by the traces It leaves behind as It flows through you. With time and attention, each of us can deepen our perception of Spirit in our lives. Among the ways of doing so are *prayer, meditation, gratitude, spiritual practices, reconnecting with nature,* and *working with spiritual counselors.*

ARE WE SPIRITUAL BEINGS?
THE NEAR-DEATH EXPERIENCE

Most of us spend our lives deluded by the belief that our traits, habits, and actions are the sum total of who we are. In actuality these characteristic behaviors make up only our conscious personalities, or the sense of self that psychology refers to as the *ego.* Our ego is the source of our thoughts, judgments, and comparisons, which usually are based on past experience or future concerns. Largely fear-based, the ego diverts our attention from appreciating the reality that exists in the present moment. We live most of our waking hours in this ego state; yet our true self, the soul (the individualized expression of Spirit), extends well beyond the limits of comprehension of the human intellect.

Letting go of the ego entails a surrender of mind and body

that most of us equate with death. The thought of our death can be overpoweringly frightful. However, it is also one of the surest methods for reconnecting with our true spiritual natures. Every experience we have of transcendence and Spirit is also one in which we feel exhilarated and access a dimension of being beyond body and mind. If death is the freeing of our deeper self, or soul, from the physical plane, isn't it possible that it, too, can be an exhilarating experience? Certainly that is the report given by the vast majority of people who have had "near-death experiences." These episodes, also known as NDEs, involve people who were considered clinically dead in emergency or operating rooms, or at the scenes of accidents, and were subsequently resuscitated. In almost every case, these people report experiencing profound feelings of peace and unconditional love, as well as a reluctance to leave the spiritual dimension to return to their bodies. They also report much less fear of death and a greater appreciation for life.

The consistency of the reports of NDEs confirms the observation of many physicians and researchers who have scientifically studied the phenomena of death and dying that the soul remains intact beyond the death of the body. One of the leaders in this field is Elisabeth Kübler-Ross, M.D., who has pioneered this investigation for most of her professional career. After nearly thirty years of scientific research, she has concluded that "death does not exist . . . all that dies is a physical shell housing an immortal spirit." She also describes the time that we spend on earth as but a brief part of our total existence, and teaches that *to live well while we are here means to learn to love*—which is an active recognition, engagement, and appreciation of Spirit in ourselves and others. In one of her studies of more than two hundred people who had experienced a near-death experience, almost all reported that they went before God and were asked the question "How have you expanded your ability to give and receive love while you were down there?"

Whether or not you choose to believe the data being gathered in the fields of thanatology and NDE, there is mounting evidence strongly suggesting the existence of Spirit beyond the realms of mind and body. Choosing to believe this theory can heighten your creativity, enhance your healing capacity, free you to realize your life's purpose, diminish the level of fear in your life, and release the self-imposed limitations of past traumas. By becoming more aware of your soul—that part of yourself that does not die—you will be better able to take risks and pursue the dreams of your life.

6. PRAYER

The most common form of spiritual exercise engaged in by most Americans is prayer. Nearly 90 percent of us pray, and 70 percent of us believe that prayer can lead to physical, emotional, or spiritual healing. Most people who pray have a greater sense of well-being than those who don't, and, when polled, the majority of people who pray say that through prayer they experience a sense of peace, receive answers to life issues, and have even felt divinely inspired or "led by God" to perform some specific action. Interestingly, people who experience a "sense of the Divine" during prayer also score the highest on ratings of general well-being and satisfaction with their lives.

In recent years, a great deal of scientific study has focused on the beneficial effects of prayer. Among the studies is one by the National Institute of Mental Health in 1994, which examined nearly three thousand North Carolinians and found that those who attended church weekly had 29 percent less risk of alcoholism than those who attended less frequently. In the same study, the risk of alcoholism decreased by 42 percent among those who prayed and read the Bible regularly. Another NIMH study conducted in the same year found that frequent churchgoers also had lower rates of depression and other mental problems.

An examination of 212 medical studies examining the relationship between religious beliefs and health by Dale Matthews, M.D., associate professor of medicine at Georgetown University, found that 75 percent of the studies showed health benefits for those patients with "religious commitments." Among patients with hypertension, regular prayer reduced blood pressure in 50 percent of all cases.

Among the pioneers in the study of the physiological effects of prayer and meditation is Herbert Benson, M.D., a Harvard cardiologist. In 1968, Benson began studying people who regularly practiced transcendental meditation (TM). The subjects meditated by focusing on a mantra, such as *Om,* that had no apparent meaning to its user. Benson discovered that repetition of the mantra resulted in a lower metabolic rate, slower heart rate, lower blood pressure, and slower breathing. He dubbed this physiological effect the *relaxation response* (RR). Benson then turned his attention to Christians and Jews who prayed instead of meditating, instructing them to repeat religious phrases such as the first line of the Lord's Prayer, "Hail Mary, full of grace," "The Lord is my shepherd," or "Shalom." He found that the phrases all produced the same relaxation response that is triggered by meditation, and that the degree of physiological benefit is determined by the degree of faith on the part of the person praying.

Since 1988, Benson and psychologist Jared Klass have been conducting a series of programs at the Mind/Body Medical Institute at New England Deaconess Hospital, inviting priests, rabbis, and ministers to investigate the spiritual and health implications of prayer. In their studies, a psychological scale developed by Benson and Klass for measuring spirituality is employed. People scoring high in spirituality—defined by Benson as a feeling that "there is more than just you" and as not necessarily religious—score higher in psychological health. They also:

- were less likely to get sick, and were better able to cope if they did
- had fewer stress-related symptoms
- gained the most from meditation training
- showed the greatest rise on a life-purpose index
- exhibited the sharpest drop in pain

To begin the practice of prayer, start with any prayer you are comfortable with or recall from your religious training as a child. You can also use a favorite psalm or passage from the Bible or prayer book you find especially meaningful. In addition, you can engage in personal prayer, talking to God as if you were speaking to your best friend. State your need or concern and ask for God's help. (It is more effective to pray for the peace that would result from having what you desire, than pray for the specific things themselves.)

In an experiment performed by the Spindrift organization in Lansdale, Pennsylvania, the effectiveness of directed and nondirected prayer was tested. Those practicing directed prayer had a specific goal, image, or outcome in mind, while nondirected prayer is an open-ended approach in which no specific outcome is held in mind. The practitioner of nondirected prayer does not attempt "to tell the universe what to do." The results proved conclusively that chances are much greater for attaining the desired outcome when one prays for "what's best"—"Thy will be done." Whichever form of prayer you choose, try to establish a regular routine and repeat your prayer morning and night.

6. GRATITUDE

I include *gratitude* and *prayer* together as number 6 in my list of the *essential 8 for optimal health*. Most religious traditions prescribe specific prayers or grace before meals as a way of thanking God for our food and sustenance. As with other spiritual practices, there is something to be gained from these rituals or they wouldn't have survived for thousands of years. A sense of gratitude for all the other areas of our lives can elicit similar life-enhancing benefits.

Gratitude has been called the "Great Attitude." Although most of us tend to take our lives for granted, they are in fact a gift, and every day that we are alive each of us receives many blessings. Even times of pain and fear, such as asthma, can be seen as opportunities for growth for which we can be grateful.

An attack of wheezing can at times be so terrifying that the asthmatic may feel as if he or she is dying, or even experience a near-death episode. Although this usually results in a greater level of general anxiety, it is possible for this individual to develop a far greater appreciation of life. By committing ourselves to becoming more aware of our blessings, we strengthen our connection with Spirit and are able to better recognize the wisdom and intelligence that underlie all of creation.

Once we allow ourselves to appreciate the lessons presented during times of struggle or life crises, the brunt of the pain subsides and a state of inner peace follows. This is especially true of most chronic diseases, which can be seen as external reflections of inner (emotional and/or spiritual) pain. Typically, when people choose to consciously focus on the positives in their lives and express gratitude for them, more positive things start to happen. For instance, while you're learning to live with your asthma, suppose you spent time each day focusing on the blessings and the many pleasures your body has provided you with in the past along with the multitude of basic functions for which it still serves you well. These include the ability to enjoy eating, drinking, digesting, eliminating, making love, and even breathing (most of the time). You may not have the ability or energy to exercise as you once did, but you can still relish the peacefulness of a quiet walk in nature. You've still retained the capacity to choose your beliefs and attitudes, as well as to experience, express, and accept all of your feelings. In addition, this physical disability can serve as a powerful catalyst for becoming better acquainted with your soul and Spirit. You may have never recognized the spiritual being that you truly are, or your purpose for being here, had you not been blessed with asthma. This may sound unreasonable or even irrational to you, but it was certainly helpful to me in curing my chronic sinusitis. For many years I suffered and felt as if I were cursed. I angrily asked of God, "Why me? What have I done to deserve this misery?" Yet now I can clearly see how this physical pain has so enriched my life. It's taught me how to give and receive love—to nurture my body, home and work environments, mind, emotional body, intimate relationships, and my soul. This is the essence of the work I came here to do, and it has become my full-time job. I call it training to thrive, and at 54, I'm healthier and more fit physically, mentally, and spiritually than I've ever been. Who knows what my life would have been like had I not been blessed with sinusitis, or yours without asthma?

Gratitude can produce powerful feelings of joy and self-acceptance, and is an attitude that anyone can choose to have, just as you can choose to see the glass half full or half empty. By focusing on what you do have instead of what you lack, you feel a sense of abundance that makes your problems seem much less acute, and you are better able to let go of negative thoughts and attitudes. This usually isn't easy to do, especially if you are feeling a great deal of fear or anger. But if you make the effort to release these painful emotions and *choose the attitude of gratitude,* even for a moment, wonderful things can happen.

Like any habit, that of recognizing and acknowledging the gifts in your life requires practice. One simple way to begin feeling grateful is the following visualization taught by Rabbi Mordecai Twerski, the spiritual leader of Denver's Hasidic community. As soon as you wake up each morning, before you get out of bed, close your eyes and picture a person, scene, or situation that made you happy to be alive and for which you are still grateful. You never would have had that experience if you weren't alive, and by allowing yourself to reexperience it, you open yourself up to the awareness that something equally wonderful can happen today. Create the habit of practicing this visualization each morning upon awakening and you will soon instill in yourself a new attitude of anticipation and appreciation for the day ahead.

Another way to cultivate feelings of gratitude is by making a *gratitude list.* This exercise is best performed before going to bed, as a way to detach yourself from any concerns or problems you may have in order to appreciate the gifts and lessons that came your way during the day. Some people prefer to write out their list; others simply close their eyes and mentally review their days, making themselves aware of all the things that happened for which they feel grateful. Either way works well. Complete the exercise by praying silently, giving thanks for all that you experienced and learned that day.

By making gratitude a regular part of your daily experience, you set the stage for living more deeply connected to Spirit. In the process, your life will be transformed into an increasingly joyous adventure.

MEDITATION

In the West, meditation has primarily been studied for its mental, emotional, and physiological benefits, while in the East it has primarily been used for thousands of years to still the mind in order to heighten awareness and contact soul and Spirit. During meditation, practitioners enter into a neutral emotional state, becoming a witness to their passing thoughts and feelings as they move into a state of heightened attention that can ultimately result in pure awareness.

As with prayer, there are many ways to meditate. Meditation can be performed while sitting or in a supine position, or while on the move—walking, jogging, and even during sports. What all forms of meditation have in common is a focusing on the breath and an emptying of the mind of thought. With regular practice, meditators typically report increased feelings of calm and peace, improved mental functioning and enhanced powers of concentration, and a deeper connection to Spirit, which is often perceived as a quiet, inner voice guiding them in their actions. Other reported benefits include increased equanimity toward, and detachment from, life events; increased energy and joy; feelings of bliss and ecstasy; and increased dream recall.

It is best to learn meditation under the guidance of a qualified instructor, but a variety of books and audiotapes are also available on the subject. The simplest method of meditation is to sit in a quiet place, resting comfortably in a chair, with your spine erect and your feet flat on the floor. Close your eyes and begin focusing on your breathing, keeping your awareness on each inhalation and exhalation. The practice is done using belly or abdominal breathing, just as you've learned to do with the breathing exercises (see page 87). To improve your concentration, you may wish to silently repeat the word *in* as you inhale, and *out* as you exhale. Or you can repeat a word or mantra, such as *love, peace, God, Om,* or *Hu* (both latter terms are names for the Divine). Allow your thoughts to come and go without lingering on them, as if your awareness were a running stream and your thoughts were simply leaves floating by. At first you may feel deluged with thoughts. Each time you find yourself distracted, simply bring your attention back to your breathing. Eventually you may notice longer periods of silence between each thought. It may take months to quiet your mind to this extent, but with consistent practice your meditation *will* become deeper and easier. Try to sit for at least ten minutes once or twice a day, gradually working up to two half-hour sessions per day. It's important to keep your practice regular and consistent, but don't force things. If you find yourself too distracted or pressed for time, end your session until next time instead of sitting restlessly.

Walking meditation is another form of meditation that in recent years has been popularized by the Buddhist monk Thich Nhat Hanh. This means of meditation is often suited for active people who find it difficult to sit still. The goal is to focus your attention in the present by focusing on each step you take in tandem with your breathing. To enhance your experience, you can mentally repeat *With each step I take I am fully present to my surroundings.* Over time, as you practice this form of meditation, don't be surprised if you find it becomes more difficult to hurry. The more you focus on the present, the less consequence time has as you discover how profound even a simple act such as walking can be.

INTUITION

As you progress in your healing journey, eventually you will find yourself being guided by your intuition, which is often experienced as an "inner nudge" or a "still, quiet voice" speaking from within. If you are not already aware of your intuitive messages, most likely it is because your intuition is having a tough time competing for your attention. Most of the inner messages you hear come from your ego and tend to be loud, self-centered, and fear-based. Intuitive messages, by contrast, come from the heart and are usually more subtle, compassionate, energizing, and enlivening.

In order to develop your sense of intuition, you will need to slow down, eliminate distractions, and do a lot less talking. The methods provided in this chapter can help you to do so. Slow, relaxing walks are another helpful way to make contact with this inner guidance. The next step is learning to recognize when your intuition is truly speaking to you and when it is not. Learning to discern the difference requires practice. One useful method for determining if the "voice" you hear is indeed your intuition is to notice how it feels. Often intuitive messages occur accompanied by feelings of excitement or an unequivocal sense that acting upon them is "the right thing to do." People who haven't learned to trust their intuition often experience doubts or fears immediately following such feelings. "How can I be sure this is true?" "What if I'm wrong?" These and similar questions can quickly quash your inner guidance if you haven't learned to trust it.

To help you know if the messages you receive are in your best interest, experiment with the following exercise. Out loud, tell yourself something that you know to be true. As you do so, notice how you feel. Now state aloud something you know to be false. Again notice how you feel. Usually people practicing this exercise experience feelings of discomfort, confusion, even pain, in their bodies when they make the false statement, whereas they feel in alignment with the statement that is true.

(Often the sensations occur in the area of the solar plexus, with false statements provoking queasy feelings or tension.)

Allowing yourself to be guided by your intuition is ultimately an act of faith. At first, learning to trust and act on the intuitive messages you receive will involve risk. The more trust you bring to your practice, however, the easier it will be to take action. Realize, too, that sometimes the results of following your intuition may be painful. Such times are not necessarily mistakes. They can be seen as lessons teaching you how to listen more effectively. Or they may be necessary to facilitate your growth and help you to better understand the higher purpose toward which Spirit is guiding you.

SPIRITUAL COUNSELORS

Due to the many uncertainties that can be part of the spiritual journey, you may consider working with a spiritual counselor, especially if you haven't been in the habit of listening to your intuition or need help in "tuning in" to Spirit. Just as you would visit a doctor to heal your physical body, or a psychotherapist to heal mental and emotional issues, spiritual counselors can help connect you to your spiritual core. The most common resources for spiritual counseling are priests, rabbis, ministers, and other clergy. Spiritual psychotherapists, medical intuitives, clairvoyants, and spiritual healers or shamans can also be of great assistance. What these healers have in common is an ability to see beyond the boundaries of the five senses. Their services may include helping you to identify your life purpose, pointing out opportunities for your spiritual growth, or to scan your body's bioenergy field to diagnose the underlying cause of a particular health condition. Their primary value, however, lies in the assistance they can provide in helping you appreciate the meaning and lessons of your daily life, especially those that are most painful.

Because of the lack of certification in these areas, to find a spiritual counselor you may need to rely upon references from people you trust, experience some trial and error, and call upon your own intuition. Keep an open mind and see how you respond to the information provided. Some of these counselors are truly gifted and can provide you with information that can be a catalyst for transforming your life.

SPIRITUAL PRACTICES

Most of us have some sort of spiritual orientation, even if it is no more than what we received in childhood. Yet we often fail to realize how much some of these practices can contribute to our health. The ritual observance of *Sabbath,* for instance, can be an enormously healing experience, as it restores the sacred rhythm between work and rest. We're so busy *doing* in our society that we've forgotten how to just *be* and appreciate the delight of simply being alive. The Sabbath day is also a particularly good time to practice gratitude as you contemplate the blessings you share with those you love. Studies also reveal that those who regularly observe a weekly holy day tend to score higher in areas of optimism, stress management, and general well-being.

Fasting is another spiritual practice that is also healing (page 139). Not only can fasting have a cleansing effect upon the body, eliminating toxins while giving the organs of digestion and assimilation a rest, it can also elicit a heightened feeling of spirituality and result in the healing of old emotional wounds. In his book *Live Better Longer,* Joseph Dispenza, director of the Parcells Center in Santa Fe, New Mexico, points out that fasting can purge the emotional body of old, toxic feelings, facilitate the release of psychological patterns that no longer work for you, and "open your mind and heart to new emotional, psychological, and spiritual sustenance." (The Parcells Center is based on the work of Dr. Hazel Parcells, a scientist and naturopathic physician who, at 41, cured herself of terminal tuberculosis using fasts and other natural methods. She then went on to live a life of vibrant, robust health until she died peacefully in her sleep at age 106.)

If you are new to fasting, try a twenty-four-hour fast, selecting a day when work and other responsibilities are limited and you won't be too active. Plan for some quiet time alone and, during the final two hours of the fast, drink six to eight glass of water to help cleanse your body of toxins.

Gabriel Cousens, M.D., at his Tree of Life Rejuvenation Center in Patagonia, Arizona, has had great success in treating a variety of diseases, including asthma, arthritis, diabetes, and alcoholism, with fasting and meditation.

The potential that spiritual practices have to heal is illustrated in the case of one of my friend and colleague Dr. Bob Anderson's patients, a 64-year-old woman named Lois, who underwent the surgical removal of a very large, aggressive ovarian cancer. The procedure left her with a colostomy, and part of the original tumor was not removable, leaving hundreds of small metastases throughout her abdominal cavity. On Dr. Anderson's insistence, Lois agreed to consult with an oncologist, only to promptly reject his recommendation of chemotherapy despite the fact that remnants of her tumor remained in her pelvis and abdomen. She was convinced that her condition would be cured by her own body with God's help, and returned to Dr. Anderson to aid her in getting well. Although she undertook many initiatives, central to her program was her faith in the power of prayer and God. Each day she meditated for up to an hour and prayed numerous times.

Four months later, Lois was finally able to persuade her surgeon to remove the colostomy to restore her internal bowel function. During the course of a long and tedious surgery, hundreds of small, metastasized tumors appeared as before. Seven of them were biopsied. Three days later the pathology report showed that their cancerous characteristics were gone. Lois fully recovered and resumed an active life focused around the activities she enjoyed and her continued prayers to God. Two years later, an operation to repair an abdominal hernia revealed that her abdomen and pelvis were completely normal, with no residual cancer anywhere. Although he has no way of proving it, Dr. Anderson remains convinced that Lois's daily prayers and meditations were somehow central to her recovery.

Finding Spirit in Nature

Nowhere is the creative power of Spirit more visible than in nature. It is here that we most directly experience life's four elemental forms of energy: earth, water, fire, and air. Earth is matter in its deepest form; water represents the receptive yielding principle; fire is the transformational energy that causes matter to change form; and air is the resultant blend of these other three elements into a subtler vibration of life-force energy. In our bodies, earth is cellular matter, water is blood and circulation, fire is metabolism and energy production, and air is oxygen, the nutrient most essential for our sustenance. By regularly exposing yourself to nature's four elements—ideally on a daily basis—you will expand your awareness of how each of them is uniquely embodied within you and more fully appreciate the healing power of nature. What follows are ways for you to do so.

Earth. Spend as much time as possible outdoors in close contact with the earth. Walking is a wonderful way to do this, as are outdoor sports, bike rides in a park, and gardening. When you can, also visit the beach, woods, and mountains, and take time to notice the beauty surrounding you. The more time you spend immersed in nature, the more aware you will become of life's natural rhythms and the ways the earth retains and radiates energy.

As a society, we need to recognize that cities and other industrialized areas are in fact unnatural and can keep us from living a life of balance. Making the effort to spend time in nature can go a long way toward restoring that balance while deepening your connection with Spirit at the same time.

Water. One of the most visible forms of Spirit in nature is the flow of water as it follows the contours of the earth. Water is a receptive form of energy and is affected by the forces acting upon it. Rivers flow, for example, due to the gravitational pull caused by the gradient of the landscape. The action of water tumbling over rocks also releases a more subtle energy in the form of negative ions, which can contribute to feelings of well-being. Swimming in the ocean, lakes, or rivers provides invaluable exposure to this special form of energy. Soaking in a mineral hot spring can also provide therapeutic benefits for a variety of ailments, and can be one of life's great pleasures.

A healthy routine that anyone can adopt is bathing in warm water at least once a day. For added benefit, practice belly breathing while you enjoy a soak in the tub. This is a very effective way to connect with your body's bioenergy field, and can help heal mental and emotional upset.

Fire. Throughout the Bible and other sacred scriptures, the dominant symbols of the divine essence in human beings are fire and light, such as the tale of Moses speaking to God in the burning bush, and the transfiguration of Jesus on the mountaintop before his closest apostles. Candlelight is also common as a tool for spiritual focus in most religions. Anyone who has experienced the pleasures of an open campfire can attest to the healing properties of fire. According to Leonard Orr, the founder of Rebirthing, spending time before an open fire, including a fireplace, cleanses the bioenergy field of negative energies and can be a powerful aid in curing physical disease. For people who want to experience such benefits, Orr recommends spending a few hours each day before fire.

Fire is also an important component of the vision quests employed by Native Americans as a means of connecting to Spirit and discerning their life purpose. The ultimate source of fire energy is the sun, which provides healing and creative energy that directly or indirectly gives life to all living organisms. Regular exposure to sunlight has been linked to a variety of mental and emotional benefits, while depression, anxiety, and other mental dis-ease can occur when we are deprived of the sun's healing rays (e.g., seasonal affective disorder, or SAD). Time spent daily in the sun is a very healthy practice as long as appropriate precautions are taken, including sunscreen, hats, and long sleeves and pants when needed.

Air. Of the four elements, air is perhaps the closest expression of Spirit, so much so that the ancient Greeks equated Spirit (*pneuma*) with the wind. The most potent method of imbuing yourself with the life-force energy of air is through meditation and other forms of conscious breathing. A daily practice of these methods can significantly energize you, open you up to new levels of creativity and productivity, and make you more aware of Spirit's guidance and power flowing through you.

SOCIAL HEALTH

"No man is an island."   JOHN DONNE

COMPONENTS OF OPTIMAL SOCIAL HEALTH

Intimacy with a spouse, partner, relative, or close friend
- Effective communication
- Forgiveness
- Touch and/or physical intimacy on a daily basis
- Sense of belonging to a support group or community
- Selflessness and altruism

Our relationship with others is the crucible that most determines how spiritually healthy we are. Optimal *social health* consists of a strong positive connection to others in community and family, and intimacy with one or more people. It is often much easier to feel our connection with Spirit during moments of solitude than it is to express that connection through our interactions with others. At the same time, our relationships offer us the greatest opportunities for spiritual growth and for learning how to receive and impart unconditional love. *True spiritual health is a balance between the autonomy of the self and intimacy with others.*

The importance of social relationships, love, and intimacy with respect to health is documented in a growing number of studies demonstrating the benefits of the diversity and depth of connection to community, family, and spouse. Lack of healthy social relationships is a common denominator among patients with heart disease, particularly when accompanied by feelings of hostility and a sense of isolation. Conversely, the longevity of terminal cancer patients with long-term survival rates has been attributed to a relatively high degree of social involvement. One of the most convincing studies highlighting the importance of community showed that Hispanics, despite poverty, lack of health insurance, and poor access to medical care, are surprisingly less likely than whites to die of major chronic diseases, including all forms of cancer, heart disease, and respiratory ailments. Further, with the exception of diabetes, liver disease, and homicide, their overall health outlook is significantly better than that of whites. Some health experts, including former surgeon general Antonia Coello Novello, the first Latina to serve in that post, postulate that the reason for this stems from Hispanic culture, which promotes strong family values and frowns on health risks such as drinking and smoking. Based on a growing number of relationship studies, researchers have concluded that *social isolation is statistically just as dangerous as smoking, high blood pressure, high cholesterol, obesity, or lack of exercise.*

The primary opportunities available to each of us for improving our social health include marriage, committed relationships, parenting, forgiveness, friendships, selfless acts and altruism, and support groups.

7. INTIMACY—COMMUNICATION, RECREATION, TOUCH

Committed Relationships and Marriage

Healthy committed relationships are probably the most effective and direct method of experiencing intimacy and unconditional love, in addition to promoting physical, emotional, and especially spiritual well-being. The model for all committed relationships is marriage, usually the most challenging as well as the most rewarding of all interpersonal relationships. It is potentially our most powerful spiritual practice. If humanity's fundamental moral principle is "Love thy neighbor as thyself," its practice begins not with the person living next door, but with the neighbor with whom we share our bed.

Regardless of who your partner may be or how long you have been involved with him or her, the key to all committed relationships is **intimacy.** Think of intimacy as *into-me-see.* As you develop the skills for seeing into—and learning to appreciate—yourself, you have the opportunity to also "see into" your partner and allow your partner to see into you. Once a commitment is made, the relationship becomes greater than the sum of its parts, allowing both partners to flourish and realize their full potential as human beings. The transformation that can occur in marriage and other committed relationships is primarily a result of letting go of judgment. As you do so, you will realize that in giving more to the relationship you are ultimately giving to yourself. Studies have shown that you may otherwise be contributing to making yourself and your partner sick. Marital conflict lowers immune function, especially in women, according to researchers at Ohio State University.

Hallmarks of a healthy committed relationship include *effective communication, recreation, and touch.* Good communication encompasses the creation of a shared vision, attentive listening to each other, and the freedom to make requests so that both partners can better ensure that their needs are met. Regular intervals of fun and recreation along with daily doses of physical intimacy and touch provide the glue for most thriving relationships. If you are interested in making a deeper commitment to your relationship, you might also consider working with a good marriage counselor or other relationship teacher.

Shared Vision. A vision that you share with your partner is a way of defining your mutual goals and focusing your energy on their attainment. Lack of a vision can cause your relationship to lose direction or become stagnant. One simple but effective way to create a shared vision with your spouse or partner is to take time to individually list your relationship goals (keep them positive, short, descriptive, specific), prioritizing them in numerical order. Then begin combining lists, starting with the goals having the highest value and alternating between the two lists to form a composite vision you and your partner are both comfortable with. The resulting "mutual relationship vision" can help keep you and your partner working together toward your common goals while reducing conflict and enhancing your relationship.

Attentive Listening. Most of us are poor listeners: We *hear* what is being said, but we don't always *listen* to it. This is because hearing can be unconscious, while listening requires conscious effort. Since communication is the foundation of any relationship, and listening is a critical aspect of effective communication, it is important to get in the habit of consciously paying attention to what your partner tells you *without responding immediately.* The practice of listening can greatly enhance both intimacy and autonomy. This type of listening can be practiced as a "listening exercise." Schedule an uninterrupted forty-minute block of time in which both you and your partner speak for twenty minutes while the other person listens *without responding.* Talk only about yourself and how you're feeling, without blaming or talking about your relationship issues. There is no discussion following the exercise.

Attentive listening makes it possible for both partners to be able to talk freely and express thoughts and feelings without worrying about judgment or criticism. Focusing on what your partner is saying requires you to empty your mind of your own thoughts and concerns as you listen, thereby minimizing negative reactions. This exercise allows for a balance between intimacy and autonomy, a critical component of healthy relationships. Cultivating the habit of attentive listening will help you and your partner create a safe environment for expressing your feelings, allowing you to be more vulnerable and open with each other, which is extremely valuable for building trust, understanding, and deeper, even exhilarating, feelings of intimacy.

Requests. By committing to another person, you enter into a relationship in which you have promised to give and receive love. But since each of us is different, what feels like love to one person may not even be noticed by another. Most of us attempt to love our partners in ways that feel like love to *us,* and are surprised when they do not react as we would. A good method for eliminating this problem is simply to tell each other what feels good to you and what you want.

It can be quite a revelation when someone you thought you knew well tells you what they really *need* from you. We often expect our partners to be able to read our minds, but we really can't know what each other wants unless we are told. Refrain from general statements such as "Love me" or "Be nice to me." Making specific requests like "I would like you to buy me flowers once a week" or "I would like you to cook dinner once a week" will significantly improve the likelihood that you will get what you need. When you do, be sure to thank your partner for complying with your request. This is extremely important, since your request is usually not an easy or natural thing for your partner to do. Otherwise you probably wouldn't have had to ask for it in the first place.

Having Fun Together. Life's daily pressures and responsibilities make it difficult to remember to have fun. For many couples, the glue that reinforces their relationship is the memory of the enjoyment they shared during their courtship and early years together. Setting aside time that you and your partner can spend in recreation together is an important way to *re-create* the joy and spontaneity that first brought you together. To rekindle some of that excitement and minimize the risk of boring routines, it helps to schedule fun activities together on a regular basis. Plan at least half a day each week to spend together away from home, taking turns each time to choose your activity. Getting out of the house, alone together, can help you focus attention on each other. Although this is more difficult to do if you have young children, it is still possible to plan an exciting evening at home after they go to bed. Choose something neither of you has tried before to add another dimension of adventure to your play, and, if you can manage it, plan several weekends per year out of town. This can be especially rewarding if a real vacation isn't feasible. Having fun regularly with the person you love is refreshing and invigorating, and can help ensure that your relationship remains healthy and fulfilling.

Touch

Touch is not only one of our most effective healing modalities, it might well be the most powerful and direct means of conveying love. The lack of touch and physical affection is being recognized as a contributing factor in causing asthma, while massage has been shown to improve pulmonary function in children with asthma. According to Saul Schanberg, M.D., Ph.D., a professor of pharmacology and biological chemistry at Duke University, "Humans need to touch and be touched, just as we need food and water." His research and that of other experts was cited in *Hands-On Healing,* edited by John Feltman.

- In a study involving forty premature infants, half of them were gently stroked for forty-five minutes a day; the other twenty were not. Although all were fed the same amount of calories, after ten days the touched babies weighed in 47 percent heavier than the unstimulated group. The stroked babies were also more active, more alert, and more responsive to social stimulation.
- When a person's wrist is gently held by someone else, the heartbeat slows and blood pressure declines.
- Children and adolescents hospitalized for psychiatric problems show remarkable reductions in anxiety levels and positive changes in attitude when they receive a brief daily back rub.
- The arteries of rabbits fed a high-cholesterol diet and petted regularly had 60 percent less blockage than did the arteries of unpetted but similarly fed rabbits.
- Rats that were handled for fifteen minutes a day during the first three weeks of their lives showed dramatically less cell deterioration and memory loss as they grew old, compared with nonhandled rats.

In a study published in July 2000, Fijian women were found to have the lowest incidence of breast cancer of any country in the world. This was attributed to the practice of breast massage, which all Fijian girls are taught as they reach childbearing age.

Yet, in spite of the mounting evidence and healthy reasons to touch and be touched by other human beings (and from the Fijian study, even by ourselves), Americans indulge very little in this simple pleasure. One study in the 1960s noted the number of touches exchanged by pairs of people sitting in coffee shops around the world. In San Juan, Puerto Rico, people touched 180 times an hour; in Paris, France, 110 times an hour; in Gainesville, Florida, 2 times an hour; and in London, England, the pairs never touched. The implications and possible causes of this phenomenon would entail a lengthy discussion, although I am sure the puritanical legacy of associating touch with sex has had a profound effect on American attitudes. William E. Whitehead, Ph.D., an associate professor of medical psychology at the Johns Hopkins University School of Medicine, believes that a significant part of the blame lies with the father of modern-day psychology, Sigmund Freud. "Freud encouraged austerity in dealing with children. And parents bought into that behavior," says Dr. Whitehead. People who aren't cuddled a lot as kids, he adds, tend to develop into nontouching adults. The cycle then repeats itself, generation after generation.

As an osteopathic physician, I learned very early in my medical training about the therapeutic value of the "laying on of hands." Although almost all of our courses and textbooks were the same as those used to train allopathic medical doctors (M.D.s), we were also taught a holistic approach to health care that included osteopathic manipulative therapy. Soft-tissue stretching (somewhat similar to massage) and adjustments or corrections in the position of the spine and other body parts (similar to chiropractic adjustments) are part of this therapy. It has taken me a while to realize that patients responded well to this treatment not only because of the prescribed techniques but also because of the healing potential of the touch itself. It is now apparent that touch is not only helpful in treating asthma, but for most other chronic conditions. There are a number of therapies in which touch is the primary healing ingredient. They include acupressure, chiropractic, craniosacral therapy, healing touch, Hellerwork, various types of massage, physical therapy, reflexology, Rolfing, therapeutic touch, and the Trager approach. If you are interested in experiencing a hands-on healing technique, I suggest trying a practitioner of one of these therapies. And if you're not so inclined, it isn't necessary to enjoy the benefits of touch by visiting a professional practitioner. In the study demonstrating the benefits of massage on children with asthma, it was the parents who performed the massage. I don't think most of us require a great deal of instruction on hugging or how to administer a loving touch. *Physical intimacy, including affection, strokes, and hugs, are a cornerstone of healthy relationships.*

Touching with love need not be sexual, nor must it be given or received from another person to be beneficial. Animals are perfectly fine sources of tactile comfort, says Alan M. Beck, Sc.D., director of the Center for the Interaction of Animals and Society at the University of Pennsylvania. Numerous studies, he adds, "definitely show that petting an animal can lower one's blood pressure." Other doctors suggest that there are health benefits to be had even from cuddling inanimate objects—teddy bears, for instance. If you have neither a pet nor a favorite stuffed animal, my prescription for helping to maintain your social health is to get several hugs daily!

There is no question that we have become too distant from one another. At a time when there are more of us than ever before (280 million), many holistic physicians and health care practitioners believe that loneliness may be Americans' greatest health risk. The recent trend toward more touching is our culture's attempt to restore a sense of wholeness and balance, and return to the norms and values of preindustrialized society. Most primitive cultures are very touch oriented. I have lived with one native group in which touch is the traditional primary mode of healing. These people believe that their healers have a gift bestowed by God, and that the healing energy that flows through the healer to the patient is God's love. Whatever its source, the healer's touch works quite well for a variety of ailments. By our standards these high-touch people might be considered primitive or underdeveloped, but they are clearly much healthier than most Americans in body, mind, and spirit.

Sex

Of all the major world religions, the Judeo-Christian tradition is the only one that does not commonly recognize the potential that sexual intercourse has as a pathway to Spirit. Other religions, including Hinduism, Buddhism, Islam, and Taoism, as well as the spiritual traditions of Africa and the Amerindians, freely acknowledge that sex, properly entered into, can be a powerful spiritual experience capable of transforming consciousness and enhancing physical and emotional health. In the West, perhaps the most well-known of these teachings on sex is *tantra*. This is an ancient system of sexual and sensual techniques for consciously controlling the mind, increasing life-force energy, and tapping into Spirit. Tantra's erotic practices include specific positions, breath, and visualization to heighten sexual energy and move it upward along the spine in order to create rapturous waves of blissful energy that can ultimately lead to enlightenment. Many mystic writings, such as the verse of the Sufi poet-saint Rumi, also refer to the Divine using the language of sex and romantic love, often equating God with the Beloved while yearning to experience union with the Absolute.

To experience sex from this exalted perspective requires expanding your focus beyond physical gratification and genital orgasm, into an experience of yourself and your spouse or lover as expressions of Spirit-in-the-flesh. Adopting this attitude leaves you extremely vulnerable and simultaneously in touch with your own divine power. Lovemaking in this state is free of the machinations of ego and proceeds slowly, gently, and consciously, ensuring that the needs of both partners are always met before moving on to the next cycle of pleasure and awareness. Couples who master this approach are able to remain in a state of heightened excitation for several hours, prolong and intensify orgasm, and experience total-body orgasms. Among the experiences they report are a continuous flow of energy throughout their bodies, a joined climax of body and soul, the sensation of being united with the cosmos, and, afterward, being refreshed and revitalized. The primary goal of "spiritual sex" isn't prolonged orgasm, however, but an experience of being more deeply connected with the person you love and, through that connectedness, an awareness of your integral role within the whole of creation. Not everyone will feel the need to master, or even explore, a tantric approach to sex; yet all of us can benefit from more-conscious lovemaking. Of all the spiritual practices, it is certainly the most pleasurable and potentially the most intimacy-enhancing. (To learn more about the tantric approach to sex, see *The Art of Sexual Ecstasy* by Margo Anand.)

Parenting

Parenting is easily one of life's most enriching experiences and, at the same time, one of our most challenging jobs. Through their children, parents have the opportunity to reconnect with play, to feel more in touch with their own "inner child," to experience selflessness, and to learn how to love unconditionally. Those of us who are parents are also provided with a wonderful forum for practicing forgiveness, trust, acceptance of ourselves and others, self-awareness, and, most of all, patience (as any parent of a teenager well knows). Perhaps the greatest human expression of love is that of parents for their children.

Unfortunately, in our society parenting isn't always consciously approached. If you are already a parent, however, it is not too late to meet your parental obligations more consciously than you may currently be doing. One useful guideline is to regularly ask yourself: *Will this action (response, activity, demand) of mine help my child's self-esteem?* One principle holds as true in parenting as it does in marriage: *To love another is to help that person better love him- or herself.* This commitment will not only affect your child's happiness in the present but will significantly impact his or her future health. In the landmark Harvard Mastery of Stress Study, college students rated their parents on their level of parental caring. Thirty-five years later, 87 percent of those who rated both parents low on parental love suffered from a chronic illness, whereas only 25 percent of those who rated both parents high in caring had a disease.

In the field of family therapy, the family is usually seen as a "system." This view holds that if a family member's behavior is harmful to himself or others, the problem and the solution lie not only within the individual but within the entire family system. This perspective encourages parents to examine their roles and the responsibility they share with their child for his or her problem. Often, a child's crisis serves as a mirror reflecting an imbalance in his or her individual system as well as in the family system as a whole. As we're beginning to learn, the crisis of asthma may represent a family dysfunction and can benefit sig nificantly from family counseling. Parents of asthmatic children, most of whom come from dysfunctional families themselves, almost always are in need of counseling and instruction with bonding exercises. One of the significant advantages of family therapy is that change often occurs more rapidly than in individual psychotherapy. In much the same way that holistic medicine treats the entire person, not simply physical symptoms, the family-systems approach recognizes the need for family therapy when any family member is suffering—emotionally or physically. If this is a situation that applies to your family, family counseling is strongly recommended. The family-systems approach is practiced predominantly by social workers.

Good parenting requires both *time* and *consistency* in order to impart the values that you would like to instill in your children. Putting in time as a parent includes being with them on a regular basis and making an effort to get to know them better. What are their talents? What do they enjoy doing? What are they thinking about and how do they feel? Learning the answers to such questions can pay big dividends for both you and your children. In fostering their growth as individuals, it is essential to give them greater power and responsibility by allowing them to make some of their own decisions. Many asthmatic children feel overly dependent on excessively controlling and smothering parents. By allowing your child to participate to a greater extent in decision making, you will also instill confidence and trust, both in themselves and in you.

Other ways to spend time as a family are to worship together each week at church or synagogue and to designate a regularly scheduled time during the weekend for a fun activity. Take turns allowing each member to choose the activity for the day. It can be a powerful confidence-builder. My adult daughters still talk about the family bike rides when, shortly after learning to ride two-wheelers, they would lead the four of us on a route of their choosing. The value of such play cannot be overemphasized. Having fun together as a family strengthens the bonds of love between each family member and defuses whatever stress or other problems may have built up during the week. Even if you cannot be with your child daily (due to being away on business or divorce, for instance), spending consistent time with them on a regular basis will help them experience the world and live their lives with the security, confidence, and caring that comes from their knowing that you love them. Remember that many asthmatic children feel an acute sense of loss, most often from an absentee father. Despite all of its inherent struggles and perils, parenting is first and foremost an incredible gift. Appreciating that gift by regularly interacting with your children is one of the most potent means for creating community and fostering both spiritual and social healing that you will ever have.

8. FORGIVENESS

"To err is human; to forgive, divine." ALEXANDER POPE

I have saved the most challenging but probably the most powerful of the *essential 8* for last. The practice of forgiveness can generate profound health benefits. Intimate relationships and unconditional love cannot exist without forgiveness. How often do you blame yourself for your past actions and mistakes? How often do you blame others for your own problems, stress, or slights (both real and imagined) against you? Forgiveness cancels the demands that you or others *should* have done things differently. Hanging on to these demands changes nothing but keeps us under stress. Refusing to forgive yourself or others keeps you locked into limiting patterns from your past, unable to mobilize the creative power in your life here and now.

The next time you find yourself blaming others, physically point your index finger at them or their images and take a look at where the other three fingers of your hand are pointed. Right back at you! Forgiveness, therefore, begins with accepting responsibility for the role you play in shaping your life's experiences. Only after you begin to forgive yourself can you truly forgive others.

A key first step in your journey of forgiveness is the recognition that you are always doing the best you can at any given moment, in accordance with your awareness at the time. This is true of everyone else as well. All of us make mistakes, and all of us ideally learn from them. You may even choose to believe that there are no mistakes, only lessons. In that moment your action or behavior was based upon past experience, environment, and heredity. You can, however, consciously choose to be different in the future. To continue to blame yourself or someone else for something that occurred in the past is energy-depleting and keeps you from moving forward with your life.

Forgiving yourself may be your greatest challenge. No doubt there are a number of things in your past that you regret or for which you feel shame. (For me, parenting mistakes have been the most difficult to forgive.) But wouldn't it be healthier to look at what you can learn from your mistake or painful lesson so that it's not repeated; forgive yourself unconditionally for not knowing more or not performing well enough; and be grateful for this opportunity to learn to do better or change your behavior? A tennis player who misses a shot he thinks he should have made will lose his confidence and ultimately his match if he doesn't quickly recognize what he did wrong, forgive himself, and move on to play the next point. Similarly we lose the ability to focus and do as well as we know we are capable of doing in the present if we do not forgive ourselves and let go of the past.

The more you are able to do this for yourself, the better you will be able to forgive others. *Remember, you are forgiving the actor, not the action.* You are not condoning cruelty, insensitivity, or incompetence; you are forgiving the offending person. By doing so, you are freeing yourself to move out of the past into the healing present. Anger is the problem; forgiveness is the solution.

Bear in mind, however, that the people you decide to forgive may not choose to accept your forgiveness. Although their refusal to do so can be hurtful, their choice should be respected. What matters is that you are taking the step to heal the relationship. The act of forgiveness takes place within your own psyche, and the person you are forgiving may therefore be totally unaware of your action. Or you may be forgiving someone who is deceased. Be realistic and don't set your sights too high: Begin with someone who has been critical of you or guilty of another relatively minor offense. Forgiving others does not necessarily mean that your relationship with them will change, but forgiving them will enable you to feel a greater sense of wholeness. Your relationship with the people you forgive may remain the same on the surface, but it doesn't mean that healing hasn't taken place. You will know it when you feel it.

Friendship

A 1997 study from Carnegie Mellon University in Pittsburgh found that people with a greater diversity of relationships were less likely to get colds. Those with six or more social ties (family, friends, coworkers, neighbors, etc.) were four times *less* susceptible to colds than those with one to three types of relationships. Researchers found that it was not the number of people in the social network that was the important factor, but the diversity. To varying degrees, most of these types of relationships can be called *friendships.*

As children and teenagers, most of us had a number of friends with whom we enjoyed sharing the day's adventures. Our friends helped us meet such challenges as each new year at school, sports, puberty, dating, family problems, and the existential concerns through which all of us passed during our journey into adulthood. Between kindergarten and college, sustaining friendships was made easier by the fact that our friends provided us with a sense of belonging, a feeling of "being in this together," and offered us a forum in which to mutually discuss the problems and issues we faced at the time. Because of such friendships, many people regard the times they spent in high school and college as the happiest days of their lives. Once past college, as they entered the workforce, got married, and juggled the responsibilities of their careers and families, a large segment of our society has lost track of their friends from the past and have not replaced them with new friends.

While most adults enjoy the company of neighbors, coworkers, and other acquaintances, by the time we reach our thirties, studies reveal that those of us who still have a best friend in whom we can confide are exceptionally rare. This is particularly true of men who, because of this lack of a confidant, experience feelings of isolation and absence of support, no matter how fulfilled they may otherwise be in their personal lives and careers.

If you find yourself in need of a good friend, realize that it's never too late to rekindle old friendships or to make new ones. All that is required is a willingness to take risks and make the effort. Having a close friend you can talk to from your heart can provide many additional blessings in your life and deepen your connection with Spirit.

Selfless Acts and Altruism

Remember a time when you stopped to spontaneously help someone, either a friend or a total stranger. Such selfless acts of giving go to the essence of Spirit, which is always with us, supporting our lives while asking for nothing in return. *Sharing with others your time, help, and special gifts and talents in ways* that benefit them provides you with perhaps the most powerful means of engaging and expressing Spirit and enhancing social health. The opportunities for sharing are abundant and may include donating clothes or money to worthy charities, volunteering time at a homeless shelter, soup kitchen, or after-school tutoring program, or simply setting aside our own tasks and concerns to address the needs of our spouses or children. (There is a great deal of truth in the adage "Charity begins at home.") Another form of sharing that is regaining popularity is *tithing.* Dating back to biblical times, tithing is the practice of donating a certain percentage (usually 5 to 10 percent) of one's yearly income to charity. Interestingly, many people who adopt the practice of tithing also find that their incomes actually begin to increase, although that should not be your motivation for doing so. However you choose to perform selfless acts, remember that the truest form of giving is one that does not call attention to the giver. As Jesus instructed in the Gospel of Matthew, "When you give to the needy, do not announce it with trumpets." The purpose of sharing is *to share,* not to acquire praise or honors. Sharing selflessly will deepen your awareness of how abundantly Spirit is giving to you.

The late Hans Selye, a pioneer in modern stress research, thought that by helping people you earn their gratitude and affection, and that the warmth that results protects against stress. Today, Selye's belief is borne out by mounting evidence that selfless acts not only feel good but are healthy. Epidemiologist James House and his colleagues at the University of Michigan's Survey Research Center studied more than 2,700 men in Tecumseh, Michigan, for almost fourteen years to see how social relationships affected mortality rates. Those who did regular volunteer work had death rates two and one half times lower than those who didn't. The highest form of selfishness is selflessness. When we freely choose to help others, we seem to get as much as—or more than—what we give.

The closer our contact with those we help, the greater the benefits seem to be. Most of us need to feel that we matter to someone, a need that volunteer work can fulfill. There is a growing number of people requiring help in our society, including the homeless, the elderly, the hungry, runaways, orphans, and the illiterate, and there are many ways to help them. Choose to do so in the way that most compels you, but recognize that altruism works best when it comes from the heart and is not calculated as a means to receive something in return.

Support Groups

As a society we are plagued by social ills, most notably divorce rates that top 50 percent, a general sentiment of feeling overworked, dual-career marriages, an increase in the number of single-parent families, and a generation of children more adrift and alone than any that has preceded them. At the same time, a movement is afoot in America toward a greater sense of community in response to the silent epidemic of isolation and loneliness that affects so many of us. As a result, there has been a significant increase in support groups for those sharing common values, experiences, and goals. Support groups for couples, divorced people, single parents, men, women, people with an illness in common (especially cancer), and people recovering from alcohol and drug addiction—and other addictions—are gathering all over the country. Many of them are affiliated with a church or synagogue, with the added purpose of enhancing spiritual growth. They meet regularly—weekly, every other week, or every month—and the participants by and large report that they benefit from the social connection they find there. If you would like to participate in such a group, most likely you can find them in your local Yellow Pages, or you can contact organizations such as your local United Way, Catholic Charities, AA group, etc. Many communities also have support groups devoted to specific diseases, and can also be found on the Internet.

Recent scientific research also verifies that support groups can play an important role in helping people with chronic disease. David Spiegel, M.D., conducted a study at Stanford University School of Medicine on women with metastatic breast cancer. All of the women received chemotherapy or radiation therapy.

Half of them were in a support group that met weekly for one year. These women lived twice as long as those who were not in a support group, and three were still alive ten years later.

SUMMARY

Your spiritual well-being is ultimately the most important aspect of your ability to care for yourself. It is also the dimension of holistic medicine that is most often neglected in our society. Becoming spiritually healthy is a process of *diminishing fear and increasing love while developing an awareness of soul and Spirit and allowing It to guide you to a deeper connection to other human beings.* This infinite source of compassionate and forgiving transcendent power is the essence of all life on earth and is the spark of life-force energy within each of us. The most direct path to becoming spiritually healthy is learning to love yourself. As you do, you will appreciate greater meaning and purpose in your life, experience gratitude for your many blessings, and become highly attuned to and trusting of your intuition. As you move beyond the confining restraints of your ego, you will become a more loving friend, spouse or committed partner, parent, and member of your community. In short, you will achieve the goal of holistic medicine: *to become whole,* and to experience a quality of life beyond anything you've probably ever imagined! Or at least beyond a score of 325 on the Thriving Self-Test.

Chapter 7

ASTHMA SURVIVAL SUCCESS STORY

There are many stories that Dr. Nelson and I could relate to you from our combined nearly fifty years of practice. I've chosen this one not only because it's an excellent example of someone who made a strong commitment to practicing the Asthma and Sinus Survival Programs, but because I feel inspired whenever I think of her. I hope you derive the same benefit from reading her story.

Jackie C. was a 52-year-old school office manager when she first came to see me in May 1992. She had been married for thirty years to an airline pilot and had two adult sons. From the age of 12 she suffered with chronic *sinusitis* and developed *asthma* in 1981. She also had multiple *allergies:* dust, grasses, smoke, perfumes, wool, and some cosmetics. For most of her adult life she'd averaged about four sinus infections per year and was treated with a course of antibiotics each time. However, in recent years the sinus disease became progressively worse, with more frequent infections, longer duration, and greater severity. During the year prior to her visit, she had experienced one prolonged sinus infection, which never completely resolved in spite of taking several prolonged (longer than one month) courses of antibiotic. It was the worsening of her condition that led her to buy *Sinus Survival*. After reading it, she called for an appointment.

Prior to that first visit she had just finished a one-month course of Augmentin (still considered the best antibiotic for treating sinusitis) and was using Ventolin (a bronchodilator, beta agonist), 2 puffs, 3 times/day; Azmacort (an anti-inflammatory corticosteroid), 3 puffs, 2 times/day; Intal (cromolyn) and Beconase AQ (a nasal corticosteroid spray), 2 sprays in each nostril, 2 times/day. During the fall of 1991 she was using the Ventolin inhaler four times a day and wrote in her medical history, "I am feeling very addicted to the asthma medication, afraid to be without it." She told her family physician that she "wanted to give up asthma medicine." After he told her this wasn't possible, she was determined to at least reduce the Ventolin. Her other goals were to improve her nutrition and her exercise program.

Her description of the months prior to her first appointment is as follows:

> I was a patient [outpatient] at the National Jewish Hospital [a center for the treatment of asthma and respiratory disease] in Denver, and with their help I was able to continue working. For exercise, I would walk around a short block, stopping several times to catch my breath, to administer medication [Ventolin inhaler], or to get my heart rate down. My husband would go with me, because he wasn't sure that I would make it back home without assistance. My problems were not obesity, but chronic sinusitis (from my teenage years) and asthma (from the early eighties). The sinus problems heightened the asthma, and the only way to combat this was to increase the strength of my medications, which included Ventolin, Azmacort, Intal, Beconase AQ, Provera, and numerous antibiotics. I had sought help from various specialists, such as allergists; ear, nose, and throat doctors; and neurologists. Two sinus surgeries in '81 and '90 had given me temporary relief, which was certainly welcome at the time, but they were definitely not long-term solutions. (The only long-term effect was decreased sense of smell.)

I was 52 years old and felt considerably older. My headaches were frequent and often severe. The constant mucus draining in the back of my throat was thick green and yellow with red blood spots, which gave me a perpetual sore throat and often affected my speech. My primary physician was concerned because I was taking antibiotics every three or four months and becoming allergic to everything he tried, which is why he finally sent me to National Jewish Hospital. It was necessary to keep Benadryl handy to treat allergic reactions to food and medications. As a result, I couldn't clean our home because of my allergic reaction to dust. I couldn't sit next to someone wearing perfume or where smokers might be present. I was constantly fatigued, sleeping twelve to sixteen hours, and never feeling as if I got enough rest. I was frightened when I'd wake up with numb hands, arms, and/or legs. There were times after my workday when I would literally crawl upstairs to bed and pray for the weekends when I could sleep longer. I often blamed my fuzzy thinking, poor performance, and graying hair on just "getting older." During this time I was extremely depressed. It wasn't a life worth living. My husband's brother, a physician, had advised him to be prepared for the worst possible outcome.

One afternoon while observing patients pull their oxygen tanks to their appointments at National Jewish, I became angry. I realized that this was my destiny if I continued under the same program. I was determined to do something to change that outcome. I told my physician that I wanted to read everything I could because I was going to find a way to get well. He agreed that I should read and become knowledgeable about asthma (I had attended numerous classes about how to live with asthma at National Jewish), but I could tell, from the look he exchanged with his nurse, that he thought I was not being realistic or practical about changing my condition. They had informed me that the asthma generally gets progressively worse for their patients who also suffer from sinus problems.

I started reading numerous books and articles and began following a diet recommended in *Dr. Berger's Immune Power Diet* to test for allergies. A friend recommended that I read *Sinus Survival* by Dr. Ivker. I couldn't believe how much he "knew about me," and I was pleased to learn that he was in Colorado. I talked with my husband about seeking his help, and he said, "What have you got to lose?" Dr. Ivker recommended that I continue with the diet, although he predicted I would have numerous allergies. At the end of Dr. Berger's test diet, I tested out allergic to everything I ate, except soy. I was equally surprised to hear Dr. Ivker say that he could take me off all my medications and cure my sinus and asthma problems. It was almost too good to be true, and I wondered how this could be possible when so many physicians had told me the opposite.

Dr. Ivker placed me on the physical aspect of the program first with environmental changes (she purchased a negative-ion generator at the first visit), vitamins and herbs (she began with vitamin C, vitamin E, beta-carotene, a multivitamin, selenium, zinc, and a combination echinacea + goldenseal), the candida treatment (candida diet, Nizoral [an antifungal medication], and Latero Flora), nasal irrigation, and a saline nasal spray. This gave me immediate, positive improvement.

At this first session, Jackie was also instructed to reduce Azmacort to 2 puffs, 2 times/day (from 3 puffs); taper off the Beconase nasal spray; and begin a very *gradual* exercise program with brisk walking, a stationary bike, or swimming. By her second visit, a month later, she reported that her energy level had increased from a 2 (a 10 is optimal) to a 5; she'd lost 15 pounds, had stopped both Beconase and Premarin, she reported she could see a difference in her breathing using the ion generator, and she looked noticeably better. She left my office with instructions to:

- reduce Ventolin to 2 puffs, 2 times/day (from 3 times/day)
- reduce Nizoral to 200mg every other day (from 1 daily)
- repeat affirmations for asthma, candidiasis, and sinusitis
- gradually increase exercise
- maintain candida diet, water intake, nasal irrigation, vitamins/ herbs

On her third office visit, about two months after the first, Jackie looked great, radiating vitality. Her energy level was averaging 7; her sinus infection was completely gone, she'd lost another five pounds and was down to her ideal body weight, she had increased the frequency of her exercise sessions, and on her occasional bad days she was beginning to become more aware of the effects of stress on physical symptoms. After this visit, she reduced both Azmacort and Ventolin to 1 puff, 2 times/day, stopped the Nizoral but continued the Latero Flora, maintained most vitamins/herbs but reduced vitamin C and garlic, made a goal/affirmation list, and began doing listening exercises with her husband.

I didn't see Jackie again for eight months, when she came in March '93. She explained that after the last visit she'd had trouble completing the assignment of the goal/affirmation list and had not returned for that reason. She had continued to feel fine until about Thanksgiving. She'd been gradually going off the diet and letting go of the irrigation and the saline spray. By mid-December she got a bad cold that became a sinus infection and her asthma got worse as a result. She decided not to take an antibiotic and had been recovering for almost three months when she came in. She still had occasional yellow mucus, energy level about a 7 on most days, and she had maintained the low dose of both Ventolin and Azmacort. She explained that she now had a clear goal—she had registered to "Ride the Rockies" in late June. (This is a one-week bike ride throughout the mountains of Colorado. It covers a distance in excess of 400 miles with a total elevation gain of close to 15,000 feet. Other than the fact that it's two weeks shorter and is not a race, it's a lot like the Tour de France, which I consider the most challenging athletic event in the world. Just to finish this ride is a monumental achievement for anyone, but especially for a 53-year-old woman who was barely able to walk around the block one year earlier.)

Jackie had already begun training for the ride, but it was a poorly defined program. She related that she had not kept up with her affirmations and had never done a listening exercise with her husband. I felt that she still had candida, although not nearly as severe a case as when she first came in, so I recommended the full candida treatment program (resumed Nizoral), helped her create several affirmations in accord with her goals, set up an exercise training regimen, and maintained the dose of both Ventolin and Azmacort.

In one month she was doing extremely well. The sinusitis was gone and her energy level was improved, but she was not able to maintain the exercise regime. Her application to Ride the Rockies had not been accepted, and she was disappointed. However, she agreed that just having been willing to take that step to apply and make the commitment was quite helpful to her healing process. She also mentioned that she was no longer taking her asthma inhalers to work with her, just using them morning and night. This was something she had always been too afraid to do in the past, never leaving the house without them. We spent much of the session discussing a recent trip home to visit her parents and the stress that generated for her. Her mother is manic-depressive, was extremely controlling during her childhood, and she feels as if she "grew up without a mother." We revised and refined her list of affirmations, then discussed anger-release techniques, and this helped her to take control of her life and make herself her top priority.

By the next session, Jackie was completely off all asthma medications (this shocked her family physician) and riding her bike regularly. She felt only one episode of chest tightness following a bike ride, and that was on a particularly windy day. She also is much more in touch with her anger and has been working on releasing it by hitting pillows against the bed. She's enjoying the affirmations.

Several weeks later she underwent minor foot surgery and had pulmonary function tests done just prior to surgery, which were perfectly normal. When I saw her following the surgery in June, she told me how pleased she was with the progress she was making with her relationships with her parents, her boss (a very controlling person), her son, and her husband.

I saw Jackie on two more occasions. The focus was on strengthening her relationships. She was so proud of herself after a recent visit home in which she was accepting and forgiving of her mother, but was also able to say *no!* To her, this was an achievement that would probably surpass Riding the Rockies.

When I last saw her in February 1994, she had not been sick with even a cold for a full year. She had continued off of all asthma medications, was taking daily maintenance vitamins, minerals, and supplements, and was maintaining a healthy diet, although not a strict candida diet. She's continued to make progress in her ongoing struggle with her boss to lighten her workload, while improving her ability to say no. She sent in another application to Ride the Rockies and needed my help to set up a training program.

I'll let Jackie describe the rest of the story:

Although I experienced immediate improvement from the physical and environmental aspects of the program, I found it necessary to complete the total program (physical, mental, social, spiritual, and emotional) to gain total freedom from my past illnesses. Under Dr. Ivker's care, my skin lost its gray hue, my hair stopped graying, and I regained my health. Much that I had attributed to "old age" was actually just poor physical health. The goal was to improve my respiratory and immune systems so that my body could care for and protect itself. This was accomplished to the degree that in 1994, I participated in Ride the Rockies, a 413-mile bike tour through Colorado's Rocky Mountains. Since then I have ridden in three more Ride the Rockies tours with family and friends.

As a result of Dr. Ivker's program, I have a life again. When I started the Sinus Survival Program, on a scale of 1 to 10, I was about a 2 or 3. Today I am in the 8-to-10 range, still taking vitamins and herbs, still working on our diet, and doing my exercises. My husband and I are making plans for our retirement which include traveling, reading, riding our bikes, visiting our children, and enjoying this beautiful world. As Dr. Ivker predicted, I no longer need to take medications for sinusitis or asthma, or for any other illnesses.

Sinus or asthma survival is not a "quick fix"; it takes commitment, dedication, time, and communication. Searching and preparing a variety of foods different from our "normal" menu, accepting that I had anger, realizing that this is a life change (not just for a day, week, or month), all required blind faith in Dr. Ivker's vast accumulation of knowledge and experience. If you are starting this program, you may struggle and wonder "Why bother, it's not worth it." Try to remember that "you are doing the best you can" and that this program is about nourishing the entire being—the mind, the body, and the spirit. Let me assure you that it is worth the effort. The Sinus/Asthma Survival Program gives you the tools you need to rebuild your body and mind and soul, which in turn gives you good health, joy, and happiness as you take control of your own life.

APPENDIX

RECIPES FOR A CANDIDA HYPOALLERGENIC DIET

NONGLUTEN GRAINS

Nongluten grains

Gluten is a protein found in some cereal grains, mainly wheat, oats, rye, triticale, barley, spelt, and buckwheat. It is responsible for making bread "springy." As the dough is kneaded, the gluten molecules join together, forming long chains that make it elasticlike.

Gluten is the major source of protein for many people who live on a wheat-based diet. However, gluten does not agree with everyone. Some digestive problems have been found to be associated with an intolerance to gluten. Fortunately, there are nongluten grains that are tasty.

Grains marked with an asterisk (*) are not recommended for a strict detoxification cleansing diet, i.e., the first three to four weeks of the Candida diet.

Gluten-free grains

amaranth, brown rice, coarse cornmeal, *millet, quinoa, wild rice

Gluten-free flours

arrowroot, amaranth, brown rice, garbanzo (chickpea), soybean, potato, *nut and seed, legume

Gluten-free pasta

Corn, *quinoa, rice, soy

Cooking Chart for Grains (in cups)

	GRAIN	WATER	COOK TIME
Amaranth	1	2–2¼	20–25 min
Brown Rice★	1	1¾–2¼	50–55 min
Buckwheat	1	2	15–20 min
Millet	1	2½	35–40 min
Quinoa	1	2	15–20 min
Teff	½	2	15–20 min
Wild rice	1	3¼	50–60 min

★Short, medium, or long grain: For softer rice use more water; for firmer rice, use less water.

RICE

If you think of a white, gummy, tasteless dish when you think of rice, think again! Whole brown rice has a pleasant, mild flavor—a somewhat chewy and satisfying texture. Rice may well be one of the easiest whole grains to introduce into your new, healthier lifestyle. Rice is extremely versatile and comes in many shapes and sizes. Here is a list to help you choose wisely:

Instant rice: Precooked rice that has had the outer coating totally removed. It lacks protein, 75 percent of its original mineral content, and most of its vitamin B.
Polished white rice: Very white, milled rice with the hull, bran, germ, and endosperm removed.
Converted rice: Rice that has been soaked and steamed before milling, to retain more of the vitamins and nutrients.
Brown rice: Rice that has had its outer husk removed. Much of the nutritional qualities have been retained.
White rice flour: Made from polished white rice, so it has little taste and low nutritional value.
Brown rice flour: Faint taste and more nutritious than white rice flour.
Rice polishings: The bran and other materials have been removed from brown rice to make polished rice.

Wild rice: Actually from the Grass family and not a true rice. It is commonly found growing wild in the Great Lakes region. It is a nutritious, tasty, and expensive food product.

Basic Steamed Rice

1 cup raw brown rice
2 cups pure water
½ tsp sea salt (optional)

If the rice looks dusty; wash it by letting water run over it in a colander or sieve. (Brown rice has a little debris left when you buy it.) Bring the water to a boil. Add the rice and allow the water to resume boiling. If you choose to, add the salt. As soon as the water is boiling, turn the heat low and simmer the rice with the lid tightly in place. Allow the rice to cook this way for about 45 minutes. Remember, by lifting the lid, steam is allowed to escape and that may disrupt the water/grain ratio.

YIELD: 3–4 SERVINGS

Rice with Snow Peas

The rice for this dish is cooked separately from the vegetables and the two are mixed together just before serving.

1 cup uncooked brown rice cooked in 2 cups of water or 3 cups of
  cooked brown rice
2 tbsp olive oil
2 cups fresh snow peas, strings removed
4 scallions, thinly sliced
½ cup thinly sliced fresh zucchini
¼ tsp sea salt
Dill, basil, or oregano to taste
¼ cup slivered almonds or sesame seeds

Cook rice. Heat oil in a skillet. Stir-fry vegetables for 3 to 5 minutes until onions are barely tender. Season with herbs, salt, and pepper. Stir hot rice into vegetables. Add almonds or sesame seeds.

YIELD: 3–4 SERVINGS

Good Mornin' Rice

> 2 cups cooked rice
> ½ tsp cinnamon
> 2 tbsp sunflower seeds
> Flax oil

Place everything except the flax oil in a small baking dish, mixing gently. Bake for 15–20 minutes in a 350°F oven. Top with a splash of flax oil and enjoy.　　　　YIELD: 3 SERVINGS

Garden Rice

> 1 tbsp olive oil
> 1 small onion, chopped
> 1 clove garlic, chopped
> 1 small carrot, chopped
> ½ cup cauliflorets
> 1 cup green beans cut in 1" segments
> ½ cup bean sprouts (optional)
> ¾ cup uncooked brown rice
> 1¼ cups water
> 2 tbsp tamari (wheat-free)
> 1 bay leaf
> ½ tsp sea salt

Heat oil in a 3-quart pot and sauté onion and garlic for about 5 minutes until tender. Add vegetables and sauté 5 minutes longer. Add sprouts, rice, water, tamari, salt, and bay leaf. Place cover on pot and cook until tender, about 40 minutes.

YIELD: 3–4 SERVINGS

Wild Rice

> 2 large stalks celery
> 1 carrot
> 6 green onions
> 2 tbsp olive oil
> 4 cups stock or water

> 1 cup wild rice
> ⅓ cup brown rice
> 1 tsp marjoram
> ¼ tsp rosemary
> ¼ tsp thyme
> 1 tsp sea salt
> Garlic to taste
> ½ cup raw almonds or sesame seeds

Chop celery and carrots in ¼" cubes. Chop green onions and sauté in olive oil. Add water and bring to a boil. Stir in remaining ingredients (except almonds). Bring to a boil, cover, reduce heat and cool for an hour or more, until rice is tender. Add chopped almonds or sesame seeds.   YIELD: 4 SERVINGS

CREAMY TAHINI RICE

> 2 tbsp water
> ½ tbsp olive oil
> 1 medium onion, chopped fine
> 1 cup mixed seeds (sunflower, sesame, and pumpkin)
> 3 cups cooked brown rice
> 1 tbsp tamari
> ⅓ cup tahini (ground sesame seeds)
> ⅓ cup water

Heat water and oil in a large skillet. Add onions and seeds and simmer for about 5 minutes or until seeds are lightly browned. Then stir in rice, tamari sauce, tahini, and water. Cook until heated through and sauce is thick and creamy around the rice. You can add 1 tbsp of flax oil before serving.   YIELD: 4 SERVINGS

MILLET

The birds of North America eat a lot more millet than do we humans. Millet is among the least familiar of the grains in our country, and it's time to change that as it is more than birdseed. Millet is a delicious, mild-flavored, yellow-colored grain. Its protein, calcium, magnesium, iron, and lecithin levels are of significant value and its versatility in recipes is exceptional.

BASIC MILLET

1 cup millet raw
3 cups water (less 2 tbsp for a fluffier millet)

Bring the water to a boil. While you wait for the water to boil, rinse the millet well, using a sieve. Add the millet and bring the mixture to a boil once again. Quickly lower the heat to a slow simmer, cover the pot, and simmer for 30–45 minutes.

YIELD: 4 SERVINGS

MILLET AND VEGETABLES

1 cup millet
1 carrot or parsnip, sliced
1 cup cabbage, sliced, or try shredded zucchini
1 cup cauliflower or broccoli pieces
1 tsp olive oil
½ tsp sea salt
½ tsp tamari (wheat-free)

Cook the millet as above until all the water is absorbed, about 25 minutes. Add the vegetables and cook for another 5–10 minutes. Add the oil and salt, and season with the tamari sauce. Serve with a green salad and flax oil dressing. For additional flavor you may add a bay leaf or some oregano to the cooking water.

YIELD: 4 SERVINGS

MILLET CROQUETTES

2 cups millet, cooked
½ cup celery, finely diced with the leaves
¼ cup carrots, finely grated
½ cup onion, diced
½ cup rice flour
¼ cup parsley, chopped
½ tsp dill

½ *tsp oregano*
Dash sea salt
½ *cup water*

Mix the millet and vegetables in a large bowl. Slowly add the salt, flour, and herbs; mix well. Add the water and mix once more. Form into small balls or patties and place on a lightly oiled (sesame or olive) baking sheet. Bake in a 350°F. oven for 25 minutes. To make the patties crispy, brush the tops with the same kind of oil after they have been baked for 10 minutes. Serve with steamed vegetables. YIELD: 4 SERVINGS

Millet Pilaf

½ *onion, sliced (if intolerant, substitute zucchini)*
1 *tsp olive oil*
½ *tsp sea salt or salt substitute*
Dash oregano
⅔ *cup raw millet*
1½ *cups water*

Sauté the onions in a small amount of water; when the onions are transparent, add the oil and simmer until soft. Add the seasonings and millet. Sauté for 3 minutes. Add the water and bring to a boil. Cover, reduce the heat, and simmer for 20 minutes. Serve with a vegetable almond stir-fry. YIELD: 4 SERVINGS

QUINOA

This interesting grain comes from the Andes Mountains and was one of the several staple foods upon which the great Inca civilization dined. Quinoa has an unusually high protein profile and expanding qualities (cooked quinoa expands to almost five times its original size). It is often a favorite with children, and its appearance is rather unique. As a cooked grain it is almost transparent, with little white O rings in the center. It can be substituted for just about any grain in recipes and has a light yet satisfying quality.

BASIC QUINOA

> *2 cups water*
> *1 cup quinoa*

Rinse quinoa thoroughly, either by using a strainer or by running fresh water over the quinoa in a pot. Drain excess water. Place quinoa and water in a 1½-quart saucepan and bring to a boil. Reduce to a simmer, cover, and cook until all of the water is absorbed (15 minutes). You will know that the quinoa is done when all the grains have turned from light beige to transparent with little white rings. Please note: Most varieties of quinoa have a naturally occurring bitter coating that helps prevent insect and bird damage. This coating is usually removed before it is shipped, but a small amount of bitter residue may occasionally remain. This can be removed simply by rinsing the quinoa before cooking. Serve with vegetables and salad for a meal.

YIELD: 3–4 SERVINGS

CURRIED QUINOA

> *2 tbsp olive oil*
> *1 clove garlic, pressed*
> *1 small onion, minced*
> *¼ tsp curry powder (or to taste)*
> *½ tsp sea salt*
> *4 cups water*
> *2 cups quinoa*

Heat a 2-quart soup pot. Add the oil and sauté garlic, onion, and then pepper. Add curry and salt. Cover and cook for a few minutes. Add water, cover, and bring to a rapid boil. Add quinoa to boiling water. Cover, reduce heat, and simmer 15 minutes. With a damp wooden spoon, mix from top to bottom. Cover and allow to rest for an additional 5 minutes.

YIELD: 5 SERVINGS

QUINOA TABOULI

2 cups quinoa, cooked
1 cup parsley, chopped
½ cup scallions, chopped
2 tbsp fresh mint (or 1 tsp dried mint)
1 clove garlic, pressed
½ tsp basil
½ cup lemon juice
¼ cup olive oil
Dash sea salt
Lettuce leaves (whole)

Place all ingredients except lettuce in a mixing bowl and toss together lightly. Chill for 1 hour or more to allow flavors to blend. Line a salad bowl with lettuce leaves and add the tabouli. Serve as a main dish salad.
YIELD: 3–4 SERVINGS

QUINOA AND PEA CHOWDER

2 cups water
¼ cup quinoa, rinsed
½ cup zucchini
¼ cup onion, chopped
1½ cups peas, fresh or frozen
2 cups water
½ tsp sea salt
¼ cup parsley, chopped

Simmer the quinoa and vegetables in 2 cups of water until tender (15 minutes). Add the second batch of water and bring to a slow boil. Season to taste. Garnish with parsley.
YIELD: 4–5 SERVINGS

AMARANTH

There is a story told that when the Spaniards invaded the Aztec people, a Spanish adviser suggested that if they wanted to crush this mighty culture, they needed first to destroy its staff of life.

This happened to be the unique and exceptionally nutritious amaranth. A decree was delivered that the cultivation of amaranth be forbidden. The ultimate demise of the Aztecs is outlined in history books. The amazing survival of amaranth, though, is a much different story. Much to the Spaniards' annoyance and amaranth's good fortune, isolated mountain villagers kept the grain alive. The grain was rediscovered and has recently made it to North American health food stores. The tiny grain has an unusual flavor and texture. Unlike other grains, it remains fairly sticky rather than fluffing up like rice. If you are a cooked-cereal fan, this grain is for you! The grain is often ground into flour and can be added to any recipe.

Basic Amaranth

1 cup amaranth
2 cups water

Bring the water to a boil. Add the amaranth, cover, and simmer over low heat for 20 minutes. For a different taste, add any spice (cinnamon, nutmeg, or cloves) or any herb (dill, basil, oregano, or curry). For a savory switch, lightly toast amaranth in 1–2 tbsp of sesame oil. Heat the oil and add the amaranth while stirring constantly over medium heat. The tiny grain will actually "pop" slightly. When this happens, add the correct amount of water and cook as described above.

Puffed Amaranth

To puff or pop amaranth, preheat a dry skillet over medium heat. Sprinkle 2 tbsp whole amaranth into the skillet. Gently stir the grain for a few seconds until it pops (amaranth doesn't pop like corn, but it does become enlarged and light golden). Quickly transfer the amaranth to a bowl and begin popping another 2 tbsp in the skillet.

RECIPES FOR A CANDIDA HYPOALLERGENIC DIET

WHOLE-GRAIN PORRIDGE

Use leftover (already cooked) nongluten grains: brown rice, millet, amaranth, or quinoa. Place the cold grain in the blender with water or nut milk. The amount of liquid determines how thick the porridge will be. Blend together to desired consistency. Heat the porridge. Add flaxseed to taste. Be creative, and after the first 21 days on the diet, try other flavorings such as cinnamon, almond butter, banana, ground flaxseeds, raisins, applesauce, or almond slivers. No two porridges are alike.

WHOLE-GRAIN HOT CEREAL

If you like Cream of Wheat, why not try Cream of Millet, Cream of Amaranth, or Cream of Quinoa? Pick any nongluten grain and grind up ½ cup in a coffee grinder. Add the grain very gradually to 1½ cups boiling water or apple juice, stirring constantly. Simmer for five minutes. Top it off with nut milk and flax oil. Also try nuts and seeds, cinnamon, applesauce, or banana slices. Quick, easy, and delicious!

NUT MILK

Place ½ cup raw almonds, sunflower seeds, sesame seeds, or cashews and two cups of water in the blender. Blend until smooth and creamy. Strain milk through a cheesecloth. Flavor with cinnamon, a dash of stevia powder, and/or alcohol-free vanilla flavoring. Delicious hot or cold, and a great milk substitute for baking.

POACHED EGGS OVER STEAMED VEGETABLES

¼ cup thin leak, sliced
¼ cup celery or bok choy, chopped
¼ cup green, yellow, or red pepper, diced
¼ cup broccoli, asparagus, or zucchini, chopped
1 large handful of leafy greens (spinach, kale, chard, etc.)

Place harder vegetables in bottom of steamer, steam for about 3 to 5 minutes, then add softer vegetable or leafy greens and turn burner off. Poach 2 eggs over easy to over medium and serve over vegetables. Sprinkle with Bragg liquid amino seasoning or sea salt.

SMOOTHIE

> *1 cup nut milk*
> *1 tablespoon organic brown rice protein powder*
> *1 tablespoon ground flaxseeds*
> *Dash of stevia powder*
> *Dash of alcohol-free vanilla*

After the first 21 days on the diet, you can begin to add other ingredients, i.e., ½ banana, ½ cup frozen berries, carob powder, etc. Be creative; blend with ice or make a hot carob drink.

SPROUTED GRAINS

Soak a nongluten grain for 12–24 hours, rinsing twice daily until tiny, ¼" sprouts begin to appear. At this point, spread the sprouts on a towel and allow to dry for 1–4 hours. Do not allow them to wither and harden. Place in refrigerator and they will last three to ten days. To serve, warm the sprouts very carefully in a pan with melted butter or soak in hot tap water for a minute or so. Eat them for breakfast or in place of cooked grains at other meals.

Sprouts are high in fiber; the enzymes in the grains have not been destroyed by the heat, and they are often less allergenic than cooked grains.

ACORN SQUASH

Cut squash in half and steam facedown for 20–30 minutes. Set in an oven dish and fill with 1 teaspoon butter or ghee. Place in 350°F oven for 10 minutes. Also delicious with flax oil, but do not add until after baking. (Avoid maple syrup or honey.)

VEGETABLE SOUP

In large saucepan, sauté diced celery carrot, zucchini, broccoli, cauliflower, cabbage, onion, and garlic in a little pure water. Cover with water and add 1 teaspoon oregano, 1 tablespoon basil, and cayenne to taste. Simmer ½ hour. Serve, then add Bragg liquid amino seasoning or sea salt to taste. Also try this soup with diced new potatoes or sweet potatoes.

Split Pea Soup
Dice and sauté carrots, celery, and onion. Boil 1 cup green split peas in ½ to 1 quart water. Add vegetables after 20 minutes. Add ¼ teaspoon thyme.

Clean Casserole
Steam zucchini and celery for 5 minutes. Turn off burner, add a good portion of mung bean sprouts, and let sit for 5 minutes. Place ½ inch of cooked rice in bottom of buttered casserole dish. Pour vegetables on top of rice and sprinkle with sunflower seeds. Bake at 350° for 20 minutes. Allow to cool slightly, then add 1 to 2 tablespoons butter or flax oil and sprinkle with Bragg liquid amino seasoning.

Curry Rice
Sauté mushrooms, onion, and green peppers in butter. Add cooked brown rice, a little Bragg liquid amino seasoning, and curry powder to taste. Garnish with fresh chopped parsley. Serve with sautéed vegetables and a side of raisins and/or coconut.

Quinoa Salad

¾ cups pure water
1 cup quinoa, rinsed 2 or 3 times
½ cup finely diced cucumber or celery
4 stems green onion, diced finely
¼ cup finely diced fresh cilantro
3 tablespoons fresh lime juice
2 tsp fresh lime juice
2 tsp flax oil
Sea salt to taste
Cayenne pepper to taste

Bring water to boil in a 1-quart pot, then add quinoa. Reduce heat and simmer, covered, for 15 minutes, stirring occasionally until grain is tender. Remove from heat and let cool, uncovered. Toss cucumber, green onion, and cilantro with cooked quinoa. Combine the lime juice, oil salt, and cayenne, and add to quinoa. Stir thoroughly with a fork to coat the grains and vegetables.

VEGGIE SANDWICH

Pile high on a nongluten bread any or all of the following: grated carrot, cucumber, green pepper, onion, sprouts, lettuce, avocado. Sprinkle with your favorite herbs and spices.

ROSE'S SAUCE

Mix together 1–2 tablespoons flax oil, 1–2 tablespoons raw sesame tahini, 2 teaspoons Bragg liquid amino seasoning, and fresh lemon juice to taste. Top steamed vegetables (cabbage, onion, zucchini, and red pepper make a great combination) and wild rice. Serve hot. This also makes a great salad dressing if you decrease the tahini and increase the lemon juice. Add your favorite herbs and spices.

CANDIDA DIET SALAD DRESSING

¼ cup fresh-squeezed lemon juice
½ cup flaxseed oil (may substitute or mix with other oil—olive, sesame, or canola)
⅛ cup pure water
⅛ tsp sea salt

OPTIONAL INGREDIENTS

Fresh or dried herbs (i.e., basil, oregano, thyme)
Curry powder
Crushed garlic
Onion powder
Sesame tahini, 1–2 tsp (will make it smooth and creamy)
Bragg liquid amino seasoning or wheat-free tamari

REFERENCES

Acupuncture

Fung KP, et al. Attenuation of exercise-induced asthma by acupuncture. *Lancet* 1986;2:1419–22.

Jobst KA. A critical analysis of acupuncture in pulmonary disease: efficacy and safety of the acupuncture needle. *J Altern Complement Med* 1995,1:57–58.

Jobst KA. Acupuncture in asthma and pulmonary disease: an analysis of efficacy and safety. *J Alt Complementary Med* 1996;2(1):179–206.

Junqi Z. Immediate antiasthmatic effect of acupuncture in 192 cases of bronchial asthma. *J Trad Chin Med* 1990;10(2):89–93.

Morton AR, Fazio SM, Miller D. Efficacy of laser-acupuncture in the prevention of exercise-induced asthma. *Ann Allergy* 1993;70:295–98.

Coleus Forskolin

Bauer K. Pharmacodynamic effects of inhaled dry powder formulations of fenoterol and colforsin in asthma. *Clin Pharmacol Ther* 1993;53(1):76–83.

Lichey, Jurgen, et al. Effect of Forskolin on Methacholine-Induced Bronchioconstriction in Extrinsic Asthmatics. *Lancet* 1984;167:25516.

Diet

Carey OJ, et al. Effect of alterations of dietary sodium on the severity of asthma in men. *Thorax* 1993 Jul;48:714–18.

Demissie K, et al. Usual dietary salt intake and asthma in children: a case-control study. *Thorax* 1996;51:59–63.

Dorsch W, Wagner H, Bayer T, et al. Anti-asthmatic effects of onions. Alk(en)ylsulfiniothioic acid alk(en)yl-esters inhibit histamine release, leukotriene and thromboxane biosynthesis in vitro and counteract PAF and allergen-induced bronchial constriction in vivo. *Biochem Pharmacol* 1988;37(23):4479–86.

Dorsch W, Weber J. Prevention of allergen-induced bronchial obstruction in sensitized guinea pigs by crude alcoholic onion extract. *Agents Actions* 1984;14:626–29.

Hoj L, Osterballe O, et al. A double-blind controlled trial of elemental diet in severe, perennial asthma. *Allergy* 1981;36:257–62.

Lindahi O, Lindwall L, Spangberg A, et al. Vegan regimen with reduced medication in the treatment of bronchial asthma. *J Asthma* 1985;22:45–55.

Ogle KA, et al. Children with allergic rhinitis and/or bronchial asthma with elimination diet. *Ann Allergy* 1977 Jul; 39(l):8–11.

Rowe AH et al. Bronchial asthma due to food allergy alone in ninety-five patients. *JAMA* 1959 Mar 14;169(11):1158–62.

Sanchez A et al. Role of sugars in human neutrophilic phagocytosis. *Am J Clin Nutr* 1973 Nov; 26(11):1180–84.

Schwarz J. Caffeine intake and asthma symptoms. *Ann Epid* 1992;2:627–35.

Schwartz J, Weiss ST. Caffeine intake and asthma symptoms. *AEP* 1992;2:617–626.

Troisi RJ, et al. A prospective study of diet and adult-onset asthma. *Am J Respir Crit Care Med* 1995;151(5):1401–8.

Unge G, et al. Effects of dietary tryptophan restrictions in patients with endogenous asthma. *Allergy* 1983;38:211–12.

Woods RK, Abramson M, Raven JM, et al. Reported food intolerance and respiratory symptoms in young adults. *Eur Respir J* 1998;11:151–55.

Woods RK, Weiner J, et al. Patients' perceptions of food-induced asthma. *Aust NZ J Med,* 1996;26(4):504–12.

Woods RK, Weiner JM, Abramson M, Thien F, Walters EH. Do dairy products induce bronchoconstriction in adults with asthma? *J Allergy Clin Immunol* 1998;101 (1 Pt 1):45–50.

Ephedra (Ma Huang)

Blumenthal M. FDA holds expert advisory committee hearing on Ma huang: Experts recommend appropriate labeling and warnings, not banning the herb. *HerbalGram* 1996;36:21–23, 73.

Duke JA, Ayensu ES. *Medicinal Plants of China.* Algonac, MI: Reference Publications, 1985.

Kasahara Y, et al. Antiinflammatory actions of ephedrines in acute inflammations. *Planta Medica* 1985;54:325–31.

Essential Fatty Acids

Britton J. Dietary fish oil and airways obstruction. *Thorax* 1995;50(Suppl):S11–S15.

Dry J, Vincent D. Effect of a fish oil diet on asthma: results of a one-year double blind study. *Int Arch Allergy Appl Immunol* 1991;95:156–57.

Heller A, et al. Lipid mediators in inflammatory disorders. *Drugs* 1998;55:487–96.

Hodge L, et al. Consumption of oily fish and childhood asthma risk. *Med J Aust* 1996;164:137–40.

Knapp HR. Omega-3 fatty acids in respiratory diseases; a review. *J Am Coll Nutr* 1995 Feb;14(1):18–23.

Lee TH, Arm JP, et al. Effects of dietary fish oil lipids on allergic and inflammatory diseases. *Allergy Proceedings* 1991 Sept/Oct;12(5):299–303.

Exercise and Breathing

Bar-On O, Inbar O. Swimming and asthma: benefits and deleterious effects. *Sports Medicine,* 1992; 14:397–405.

Berlowitz D, Denehy L, et al. The Buteyko asthma breathing technique. *Med J Aust* 1995;162:53.

Bowler SD, et al. Buteyko breathing techniques in asthma: a blinded randomized controlled trial. *Med J Aust* 1998 Dec 7–21; 169(11–12):575–78.

Buchholz I. Breathing, voice and movement therapy: applications to breathing disorders. *Biofeedback Self Regul* 1994;19: 141–53.

Fluge T, Richter J, et al. Long-term effects of breathing exercises and yoga in patients with bronchial asthma. *Pneumologie* 1994;48:484–90.

Huang SW, Veiga R, et al. The effect of swimming in asthmatic children—participants in a swimming program in the city of Baltimore. *J Asthma* 1989;26:117–21.

Jain SC, Rai L, Valecha A, et al. Effect of yoga training on exercise tolerance in adolescents with childhood asthma. *J Asthma* 1991;28(6):437–42.

Nagarathna R, Nagendra HR. Yoga for bronchial asthma: a controlled study. *Br Med J* 1985;291:1077–79.

Nagendra HR, Nagarantha R. An integrated approach of yoga therapy for bronchial asthma: a 3- to 54-month prospective study. *J Asthma* 1986;23:123–37.

Orenstein DM. Exercise tolerance and exercise conditioning in children with chronic lung disease. *J Pediatr* 1988;112:1043–7.

Schnall R, Ford P, et al. Swimming and dry land exercise in children with asthma. *Aust Paediatr J* 1982;18:23–27.

Singh V. Effect of respiratory exercises on asthma: the pink city lung exerciser. *J Asthma* 1987;24:355–9.

Singh V. Effect of respiratory exercises on asthma. *J Asthma* 1987;24:355–59.

Tanizaki Y, Kitani H, Okazaki M, et al. Clinical effects of complex spa therapy on patients with steroid-dependent intractable asthma (SDIA). *Aerugi* 1993;42:219–27.

References

Vedanthan PK, Kesavalu LK, Murthy KC, et al. Clinical study of yoga techniques in University students with asthma: a controlled study. *Allergy Asthma Proc* 1998;19(1):3–9.

Folic Acid

Bailey LB, *Folate in Health and Disease.* New York: Dekker, 1995.

Ginkgo Biloba

Guinot P, et al. Effect of BN-52063, a specific PAF-acether antagonist, on bronchial provocation test to allergens in asthmatic patients: a preliminary study. *Prostaglandins* 1987;34(5):723–31.

Kleijnen J, Knipschild P. *Ginkgo biloba. Lancet* 1992;340:1136–39.

Kose K, Dogan P. Lipoperoxidation induced by hydrogen peroxide in human erythrocyte membranes. 2. Comparison of the antioxidant effect of *Ginkgo biloba* extract (EGb 761) with those of water-soluble and lipid soluble antioxidants. *J Int Med Res* 1995;23:9–18.

Smith PF, MacLennan K, Darlington CL. The neuroprotective properties of the *Ginkgo biloba* leaf: a review of the possible relationship to platelet-activating factor (PAF). *J Ethnopharm* 1996;50:131–39.

Glutathione

Hasselmark L, Malmgren P, Ung G, Zettktrom O. Lowered platelet glutathione peroxidase activity in patients with intrinsic asthma. *Allergy* Oct 1990; 45(7):523–27.

Hydrochloric Acid

Bray, GW. The Hypochlorhydria of Asthma in Childhood. *J Nutr Med* 1990;1:347–360.

Khellin

Kennedy MC, Stock J. The bronchodilator action of khellin. *Thorax* 1952;7:43–65.

Licorice

Epstein MT, Espiner EA, Donald RA, Hughes H. Effect of eating licorice on the renin-angiotensin aldosterone axis in normal subjects. *Br Med J* 1977;1:488–490.

Ghosh D, Wawrzak V, Pletnev M, et al. Molecular mechanism of inhibition of steroid dehydrogenases by licorice-derived steroid analogs in modulation of steroid receptor function. *Ann NY Acad Sci* 1995;761:341–3.

Okimasu E, et al. Inhibition of phospholipase A2 and platelet aggregation by glycyrrhizin, an anti-inflammatory drug. *Acta Med Okayama* 1983;37:385–91.

Lobelia

Cambar P, et al. Bronchopulmonary and gastrointestinal effects of lobeline. *Arch Int Pharmacodyn* 1969;177:1–27.

Halgamagyi DJF, et al. Adrenocortical pathways of lobeline protection in some forms of experimental lung edema in the rat. *Dis Chest* 1958;33:285–96.

Mitchell W. *Naturopathic Applications of the Botanical Remedies.* Seattle: W. Mitchell, 1983.

Magnesium

Britton J, et al. Dietary magnesium, lung function, wheezing and airway hyperreactivity in a random adult population sample. *Lancet* 1994 Aug 6; 344(8919):357–62.

Ciarallo L, et al. Higher dose intravenous magnesium therapy for children with moderate to severe acute asthma. *Arch Pediatr Adolesc Med* 2000;154:979–83.

Ciarello L, et al. Intravenous magnesium therapy for moderate to severe pediatric asthma: results of a randomized, placebo-controlled trial. *J Pediatr* 1996 Dec;129(6):809–14.

Hill J, Britton J, et al. Investigation of the effect of short-term change in dietary magnesium intake in asthma. *Eur Respir J* 1997;10:2225–29.

Okayama H, et al. Treatment of status asthmaticus with intravenous magnesium sulfate. *J Asthma* 1991 Feb;28(1):11–17.

N-acetylcysteine (NAC)

British Thoracic Society Research Committee. Oral N-Acetylcysteine and excacerbation rates in patients with chronic bronchitis and severe airway obstruction. *Thorax* 1985;40:832–835.

Tattersall AB, et al. Acetylcysteine (Fabrol) in chronic bronchitis—a study in general practice. *J Int Med Res* 1983;1:279–284.

Negative Ions

Ben–Dov et al. Effect of negative ionization of inspired air on the response of asthmatic children to exercise and inhaled histamine. *Thorax* 1983 Aug;38(8):584–88.

Warner JA, Marchant JL, Warner JO. Double-blind trial of ionizers in children with asthma sensitive to the house dust mite. *Thorax* 1993;48:330–33.

Quercetin

Cody V, Middleton E, et al. *Plant Flavanoids in Biology and Medicine II—Biochemical, Pharmacological, and Structure-activity relationships.* New York: Alan R. Liss, 1988.

Foreman JC. Mast cells and the actions of flavanoids. *J Allergy Clin Immunol* 1984 Jun;73(6):769–74.

Middleton E Jr., et al. Quercetin: an inhibitor of antigen-induced basophil histamine release. *J Immunol* 1981 Aug;127(2):546.

References

Tarayre JP, Lauressergues H. Advantages of a combination of proteolytic enzymes, flavanoids and ascorbic acid in comparison with non-steroid anti-inflammatory agents. *Arzneimittelforschung* 1977;27:1144–1149.

Relaxation and Stress-Release Techniques

Alexander AB, Miklich DR, Hershkoff H. The immediate effects of systematic relaxation training on peak expiratory flow rates in asthmatic children. *Psychosom Med* 1972;34(5):388–94.

Collison DR. Which asthmatic patients should be treated with hypnotherapy? *Med J Aust* 1975 Jun 21;1(25):776–81.

Field T, Henteleff T, et al. Children with asthma have improved pulmonary functions after massage therapy. *J Pediatr* 1998;132: 854–58.

Henry M, deRivera LG, et al. Improvement of respiratory function in chronic asthma patients with autogenic training. *J Psychosom Res* 1993;37:265–70.

Kohen DP, Wynne E. Applying hypnosis in a preschool family asthma education program: uses of storytelling, imagery and relaxation. *Am J Clin Hypnosis* 1997;39(3):169–81.

Kotses H, Harver A, Segreto J, et al. Long-term effects of biofeedback-induced facial relaxation on measures of asthma severity in children. *Biofeedback Self Reg* 1991;16:1–21.

Lehrer PM. Emotionally triggered asthma: a review of research literature and some hypotheses for self-regulation therapies. *Appl Psychophys Biofeedback* 1998;23(1):13–41.

Lehrer PM, Hochron SM, et al. Relaxation and music therapies for asthma among patients prestabilized on asthma medication. *J Behav Med* 1994;17:1–24.

Lehrer PM. Relaxation decreases large-airway but not small airway asthma. *J Psychosom Res* 1986;30(1):13–25.

Luparello T, et al. Influence of suggestion on airway reactivity in asthmatic subjects. *Psychosom Med* 1968 Nov/Dec;30(6): 819–25.

Mass R, Richter R, Dahme B. Biofeedback induced voluntary

reduction of respiratory resistance in severe bronchial asthma. *Behav Res Ther* 1996;34(10):815–19.

Morrison JB. Alternative and complementary medicine for asthma. *Thorax* 1992;47:762.

Peper E, Tibbetts V. Fifteen month follow-up with asthmatics utilizing EMG/Incentive inspirometer feedback. *Biofeedback Self Reg* 1992;17:143–51.

Rider MS et al. Effect of immune system imagery on secretory IgA. *Biof Self Regul* 1990 Dec; 15(4):317–33.

Smyth JM et al. Effects of writing about stressful experiences on symptom reduction in patients with asthma or rheumatoid arthritis: a randomized trial. *JAMA* 1999 Apr 14;28(14): 1304–09.

Strunk RC. Physiologic and psychological characteristics associated with deaths due to asthma in childhood. *JAMA* 1985 Sep 6; 254(9):1193–98.

Vazquez I. Buceta J. Relaxation therapy in the treatment of bronchial asthma: effects on basal spirometric values. *Psychother Psychosom* 1993;60:106–12.

Wilson AR, Honsberger R, et al. Transcendental meditation and asthma. *Respiration* 1975;32:74–80.

Selenium

Flatt A, et al. Reduced selenium in asthmatic subjects in New Zealand. *Thorax* Feb 1990.

Hasselmark L, et al. Selenium supplementation in intrinsic asthma. *Allergy* 1993; 48(1):30–36.

Kadrabova J, et al. Selenium status is decreased in patients with intrinsic asthma. *Biol Trace Elem Res* 1996;52(3):241–8.

Vitamin B$_6$

Collipp PJ, et al. Pyridoxine treatment of childhood bronchial asthma. *Ann Allergy* 1975;35:93–97.

References

Kaslow JE. Double-blind trial of pyridoxine (vitamin B_6) in the treatment of steroid-dependent asthma. *Ann Allergy* 1993; 71(5):492.

Reynolds RD, Natta CL. Depressed plasma pyridoxal phosphate concentrations in adult asthmatics. *Am J Clin Nutr* 1985 Apr;41(4):684–88.

Sur S, et al. Double-blind trial of pyridoxine (vitamin B_6) in the treatment of steroid-dependent asthma. *Ann Allergy* 1993; 70(2):147–52.

Weir MR, et al. Depression of vitamin B_6 levels due to theophylline. *Ann Allergy* 1990;65:59–62.

Vitamin C

Anah C, et al. High dose ascorbic acid in Nigerian asthmatics. *Trop Geogr Med* 1980; 32:132–37.

Anderson R, Hay I, Van Wyk HA, et al. Ascorbic acid in bronchial asthma. *S Afr Med J* 1983; 63:649–52.

Cohen HA, et al. Blocking effect of vitamin C in exercise-induced asthma. *Arch Pediatr Adolesc Med* 1997;151(4):367–70.

Hatch GE. Asthma, inhaled oxidants, and dietary antioxidants. *Am J Clinical Nutrition* March 1995; 48(1):30–36.

Olusi SO, Ojutiku OO, Jessop WJE, Iboko MI. Plasma and white blood cell ascorbic acid concentrations in patients with bronchial asthma. *Clinic Chiica Acta* 1979;92:161–66.

RESOURCE GUIDE

For more information about the Asthma Survi\
make an appointment with Dr. Todd Nelson, p.
744-7858.

The following organizations provide information particularly
useful for people with asthma:

- Asthma and Allergy Foundation of America *www.aafa.org*
- Mothers of Asthmatics *www.aanma.org*

The following organizations offer additional information
about various aspects of the Asthma Survival Program, and provide referrals to practitioners of the many therapies that contribute to this holistic approach for treating, preventing, and
curing asthma.

Holistic Medicine
American Board of Holistic Medicine (ABHM)
Phone (425) 741-2996
Fax: (425) 787-8040

*The ABHM is the first organization to certify physicians in Holistic
Medicine (December 2000 was the first certification examination) and
to create the standard of care for holistic medical practice. Provides a referral list of board-certified holistic physicians.*

*...ion's oldest advocacy group (founded in 1978) devoted to pro-
...ng, teaching, and researching holistic medicine. Provides a list of re-
...errals nationwide of holistic physicians (M.D.s and D.O.s) (available
on the Web site).*

Osteopathic Medicine

American Academy of Osteopathy
3500 DePauw Blvd, Suite 1080
Indianapolis, IN 46268
Phone (317) 879-1881

*Affiliate organization representing D.O.s who provide osteopathic ma-
nipulative treatments and/or cranial osteopathy as part of their practice.*

Craniosacral Therapy

Cranial Academy
8606 Allisonville Road, Suite 130
Indianapolis, IN 46268
Phone (317) 594-0411
Fax (317) 594-0411 and (317) 594-9299

Provides information and a referral list of craniosacral therapists.

Upledger Institute
11211 Prosperity Farms Road
Palm Beach Gardens, FL 33410
Phone (407) 622-4706
Fax (407) 622-4771

Offers training, information, and referrals.

Acupuncture/Traditional Chinese Medicine

American Association for Oriental Medicine
433 Front Street
Catasauqua, PA, 18032
Phone (610) 266-1433
Fax (610) 264-2768

Professional association for non-M.D. acupuncturists. Offers publications and referral directory of members nationwide.

American Academy of Medical Acupuncture
58200 Wilshire Blvd., Suite 500
Los Angeles, CA 90036
Phone (213) 937-5514

Professional association of physician acupuncturists (M.D.s and D.O.s). Provides educational materials, postgraduate courses, and a membership directory of members nationwide.

National Commission for the Certification of Acupuncturists
1424 16th NW, Suite 601
Washington, DC 20036
Phone (202) 232-1404

Provides information about acupuncture and offers a test used by various states to determine competency of acupuncture practitioners.

National Acupuncture Detoxification Association
3115 Broadway, Suite 51
New York, NY 10027
Phone (212) 993-3100

Leading organization of its kind. Conducts research on, and provides training in the use of acupuncture to treat addiction, including alcoholism.

Qigong Institute/East-West Academy of Healing Arts
450 Sutter, Suite 916
San Francisco, CA 94108
Phone (415) 788-2227

Provides education, training, and research about qigong in relation to health and healing.

Behavioral Medicine/Mind–Body Medicine

National Institute for the Clinical Application of Behavioral Medicine
P.O. Box 523
Mansfield Center, CT 06250
Phone (860) 456-1153
Fax (860) 423-4512

Provides conferences and information for practitioners.

Association for Humanistic Psychology
45 Franklin Street, Suite 315
San Francisco, CA 94102
Phone (415) 864-8850

Provides publications about humanistic psychology and a list of referrals.

Center for Mind-Body Medicine
5225 Connecticut Avenue NW, Suite 414
Washington, DC 20015
Phone (202) 966-7338

An educational program for health and mental health professionals, and laypeople interested in exploring their own capacities for self-knowledge and self-care. Provides educational and support groups for people with chronic illness, stress management groups, and training and programs in mind-body health care.

Mind/Body Medical Institute
New Deaconess Hospital
185 Pilgrim Road
Boston, MA 02215
Phone (617) 632-9530

Provides research, training, and conferences related to behavioral medicine, stress reduction, yoga, and meditation.

Bodywork/Massage Therapies

American Massage Therapy Association
820 Davis Street, Suite 100
Evanston, IL 60201
Phone (312) 761-2682

Provides comprehensive information on most areas of bodywork and massage, including an extensive review of the latest scientific research. Also publishes Massage Therapy Journal, *available at most health food stores and many newsstands nationwide.*

Associated Bodywork and Massage Professionals
P.O. Box 489
Evergreen, CO 80439
Phone (303) 674-8478

Provides information and referrals.

Rolfing

International Rolf Institute
302 Pearl Street
Boulder, CO 80306
Phone (303) 449-5903

Provides information, training, and referral directory.

Reflexology

International Institute of Reflexology
P.O. Box 12462
St. Petersburg, FL 33733
Phone (813) 343-4811

Provides information, training, and referrals.

Chiropractic

American Chiropractic Association
1701 Clarendon Blvd.
Arlington, VA 22209
Phone (703) 276-8800

Professional association offering education and research into chiropractic. Also offers publications.

International Chiropractors Association
1110 North Glebe Road, Suite 1000
Arlington, VA 22201
Phone (800) 423-4690 and (703) 528-5000

Professional association offering education and research into chiropractic. Also offers publications.

Diet and Nutrition

American College for Advancement in Medicine (ACAM)
23121 Verdugo Drive, Suite 204
Laguna Hills, CA 92653
Phone (800)-532-3688

ACAM provides information about the use of nutritional supplements and a referral directory of physicians worldwide who have been trained in nutritional medicine.

American College of Nutrition
722 Robert E. Lee Drive
Wilmington, NC 28480
Phone (919) 452-1222

Information resource for nutrition research.

Center for Science in the Public Interest
1875 Connecticut Avenue NW, Suite 300
Washington, DC 20009
Phone (202) 332-9110
Fax (202) 265-4954

Provides a directory of organic mail-order suppliers, hormone-free beef suppliers, and general information on diet and nutrition.

American Dietetic Association
216 West Jackson, Suite 800
Chicago, IL 60606
Phone (312) 899-0040

Provides information and certification.

International Association of Professional Natural Hygienists
Regency Health Resort and Spa
2000 South Ocean Drive
Hallandale, FL 33009
Phone (305) 454-2220

Professional organization of physicians who specialize in therapeutic fasting.

Energy Medicine

International Society for the Study of Subtle Energies and Energy Medicine (ISSSEEM)
356 Goldco Circle
Golden, CO, 80401
Phone (303) 278-2228
Fax (303) 279-3539

Research organization; provides education and information, as well as publications.

Therapeutic Touch

Nurse Healers Professional Associates, Inc.
1211 Locust Street
Philadelphia, PA 19107
Phone (215) 545-8079

Provides information on training, conferences, and referrals of TT practitioners. Also publishes a newsletter.

Healing Touch

Colorado Center for Healing Touch, Inc.
198 Union Blvd., Suite 204
Lakewood, CO 80228

Provides information and referrals.

Reiki

Reiki Alliance
P.O. Box 41
Cataldo, ID 83810
Phone (208) 682–3535

Provides information and referrals.

Energy Devices

Tools For Exploration
9755 Independence Avenue
Chatsworth, CA 91311
Phone (888) 748–6657

Provides nonmedical energy machines and other devices. Free catalog available by request.

Environmental Medicine

American Academy of Environmental Medicine
7701 E. Kellogg Suite 625
Wichita, KS 67202
Phone (316) 684–5500

Provides referral list of physicians practicing environmental medicine, as well as a newsletter and other information.

Human Ecology Action League (HEAL)
P.O. Box 49126
Atlanta, GA 30359
Phone (404) 248–1898

Provide referrals to support groups that assist people suffering from environmental illness.

Immuno Labs
1620 West Oakland Park Blvd., Suite 300
Fort Lauderdale, FL 33311
Phone (800) 321-9197

A lab specializing in allergy testing. Also provides referrals to environmental physicians worldwide.

Herbal Medicine
American Botanical Council
P.O. Box 201660
Austin, TX 78720
Phone (512) 331-8868

A nonprofit research organization and education council that serves as a clearinghouse of information for professionals and laypeople alike.

Herb Research Foundation
1007 Pearl Street
Boulder, CO 80302
Phone (303) 449-2265

Provides research information and referrals to resources on botanical medicine. Also publishes HerbalGram.

Homeopathy
International Foundation for Homeopathy
2366 Eastlake Avenue East, Suite 301
Seattle, WA 98102
Phone (206) 324-8230

Provides training in homeopathy and offers referrals.

National Center for Homeopathy
801 North Fairfax, Suite 306
Alexandria, VA 22314
Phone (703) 548-7790

Offers training in homeopathy and provides referrals.

Laboratory

Great Smokies Diagnostic Laboratory
63 Zillicoa St.
Asheville, NC 28801-1074
Phone (800) 522-4762

Offers fully certified advanced assessments using over 100 diagnostic tests of digestive, immune, endocrine, nutritional, and metabolic function—supported by a comprehensive network of educational and scientific resources.

Naturopathic Medicine

American Association of Naturopathic Physicians
2366 Eastlake Avenue East, Suite 322
Seattle, WA 98102
Phone (206) 323-7610

Provides information, publications, and a referral directory of naturopathic physicians. Also in the forefront in licensing of naturopaths throughout the United States.

The Institute for Naturopathic Medicine
66½ North State Street
Concord, NH 03301
Phone (603) 255-8844

A nonprofit organization promoting research about naturopathy. Offers information to professional and laypeople, along with the general media.

PRODUCT INDEX

The following are all currently available through *Thriving Health Products* (toll free at (888) 434-0033 or the Web site: www. sinussurvival.com). Some of these products are also available at health food stores, pharmacies, department stores, and bookstores.

Vitamins/Herbs/Minerals/Supplements/Homeopathics

Candida-Free
Magnesium Extra (magnesium glycinate)
Super Potency Essential Fatty Acids (omega-3 oils, EPA, and DHA)
Standardized Coleus Forskolin
Quercetin with bromelain
Lobelia
Super Potency Garlic-6000
Sinus Survival Ester C
Sinus Survival Masquelier's OPC Grape Seed
Sinus Survival Eucalyptus Spray
Sinus Survival Elderberry Cough Syrup
Sinus Survival Zinc Cold Lozenges
Sinus Survival EchinOsha Blend
Professional Health Products Mycocan Combo
Life Center Intestinalis
International Bio-Tech Latero-Flora

Nasal Hygiene—*Moisture/Stream/Irrigation*

Sinus Survival Nasal Spray
Kaz TheraSteam Personal Steam Inhaler
RST Respiratory Steam Inhaler
SinuCleanse Irrigation System
SinuCleanse Saline Refills
SinuCleanse Video
Grossan Nasal Irrigator
Water Pik

Ionizers/Air Cleaners/Humidfiers

Sinus Survival "Air Vitalizer" Ionizer
Bionaire ULPA Filter Air Cleaners
Bionaire ULPA Filter Replacements
Bionaire Warm Mist Humidifiers
Bionaire Climate Check (Temperature/Humidity Gauge)
Sinus Survival Pleated Furnace Filters

Cleaning Products

DuPont Vacuum Bags
Wizard Dust Cloths

INDEX

Page numbers in italics refer to tabular information.

Index

Index

Index

Index

Index

ABOUT THE AUTHORS

Robert S. Ivker, D.O.

Dr. Ivker is a holistic family physician and healer. He began practicing family medicine in Denver in 1972, after graduating from the Philadelphia College of Osteopathic Medicine. He completed a family practice residency at Mercy Medical Center in Denver and was certified by the American Board of Family Practice (ABFP) from 1975 to 1988. For the past 13 years his holistic medical practice has focused on the treatment of chronic disease and the creation of optimal health. He is an Assistant Clinical Professor in the Department of Family Medicine and a Clinical Instructor in the Department of Otolaryngology at the University of Colorado School of Medicine. Dr. Ivker is a cofounder of the American Board of Holistic Medicine (ABHM) and cocreator of the first board certification examination in holistic medicine in December 2000. He was the President of the American Holistic Medical Association (AHMA) from 1996 to 1999. Along with the four editions of the best-selling *Sinus Survival: The Holistic Medical Treatment for Sinusitis, Allergies, and Colds,* Dr. Ivker is the coauthor of *The Self-Care Guide to Holistic Medicine: Creating Optimal Health* and *Thriving:*

The Holistic Guide to Optimal Health for Men. Asthma Survival is part of a Survival Guide series that also includes *Arthritis Survival, Backache Survival,* and *Headache Survival,* all published by Tarcher/Putnam in 2001 and 2002. He has been married for thirty-two years to Harriet, a psychiatric social worker; they have two daughters—Julie and Carin—and live in Littleton, Colorado.

Todd H. Nelson, N.D., D.Sc.

Dr. Nelson is a naturopathic doctor and director of the Tree of Life Wellness Center, Colorado's busiest naturopathic clinic. His specialty is clinical nutrition and functional medicine. He has been serving the Denver/Boulder community for eighteen years, integrating comprehensive holistic health care through balanced, educational approaches to self-care. Dr. Nelson lectures extensively on a broad range of holistic health topics, both locally and nationally. He also teaches a corporate wellness program, Stress Mastery, to major corporations. He is the cohost of a popular radio show, HealthTime on KHOW, Colorado's #1 weekly talk show on alternative health care. Todd lives in Denver with his wife, Dixie, and four daughters.